For general information on our other products and services or to obtain technical support, please contact our Customer Service department within the US at +1 (813) 640–0771 or in Europe +44 131 380 6280 or email contact@upgraders.com.

UPGRADERS® publishes its books in a variety of electronic and print formats. Some content that appears in print may not be available in electronic books, and vice versa.

Designer: Külli Tõnisson

Food Photography: Naomi Sherman

Science: Dr. Henning Sartor, PhD

Texts & Recipes: Helen Marie Loorents, MBA

Editor: Dr. Claudia Preyer

ISBN: 978 - 0 - 9908594 - 2 - 0

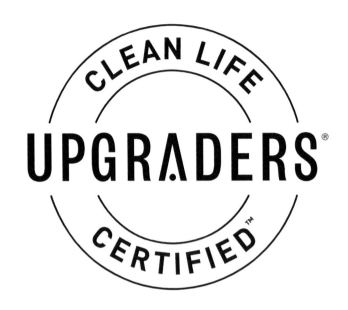

CLEAN LIFE
UPGRADERS®
CERTIFIED™

TOXIN BUILDUP – The hidden culprit behind weight gain,
health decline and premature aging.

## DETOX to UPGRADE YOUR HEALTH & BEAUTY in Just 21 Days!

Only a detoxified body can regenerate to heal,
lose weight, sleep better, look younger and thrive …

# TABLE OF CONTENTS

# I. OVERVIEW

In a world of abundance, the paradox of malnutrition and declining health becomes increasingly evident. Wrong lifestyle choices not only trigger environmental toxins and chronic digestive damage but also impact well-being and accelerate the aging process. These silent toxins, at the root of silent inflammation, contribute to a range of health issues. Our daily exposure to stressors and toxins through lifestyle, nutrition, and our surroundings intensifies as we age, amplifying the consequences. As the body ages, its ability to detox, recover, and heal diminishes, with older senescent cells outnumbering their younger, more vibrant counterparts.

To achieve optimal health, a cellular cleanse is essential. Restoring nutrient balance and enabling maximum absorption, this process empowers the body to heal, shed excess weight, improve sleep, and renew vitality.

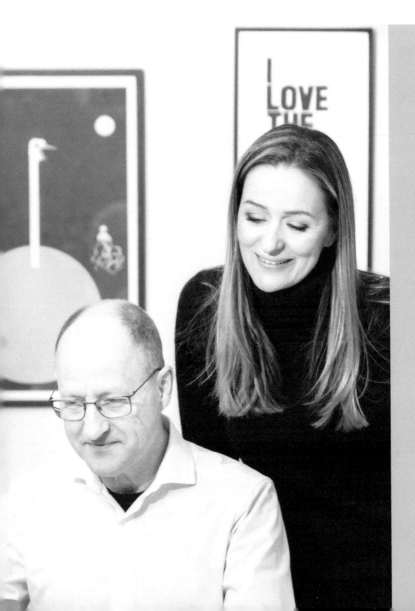

"With over 25 years of experience in healthcare and corporate America, I encountered burnout and numerous health challenges. My transformative 10-day detox at an Austrian Alps wellness clinic shed light on the profound impact of toxins on health, beauty, vitality, and mental well-being. The solution was crystal clear: embrace clean living.

Inspired by the century-old clinic detox pioneered by Austrian Dr. Franz Xaver Mayr, a method still trusted by top European wellness clinics today, we've expertly adapted this approach for home use. Guided by German microbiome and toxicity specialist, Dr. Henning Sartor, our program unlocks centuries-old wisdom to embark on a remarkable journey to better health."

*Helen Marie Loorents,*

THE FOUNDER OF UPGRADERS

# 1.1 DO I NEED TO DETOX?

The rise of industrialization has introduced a surge in toxic chemical use, infiltrating various aspects of our surroundings, from soil and food to skincare products and homes. The hectic pace of modern life exacerbates toxicity through improper eating habits and increased fermentation during digestion. These accumulated toxins hinder our cells' optimal function, leading to malnourishment. When our body's detox capacity is overwhelmed, it manifests itself as a health issue—a warning sign that detoxification is essential.

Fasting, or abstaining from food, emerges as a powerful detox method. It promotes autophagy, a process that cleans up worn-out cells, offering anti-aging benefits. During a minimum of 16-hour overnight fasting, growth hormone (somatotropin) production and autophagy are activated. Growth hormone aids in breaking down fat, building muscle, extending the life of cells, and promoting DNA repair mechanisms in the body.

The optimal detox frequency varies from 1 to 3 times per year, depending on your environment and overall health status.

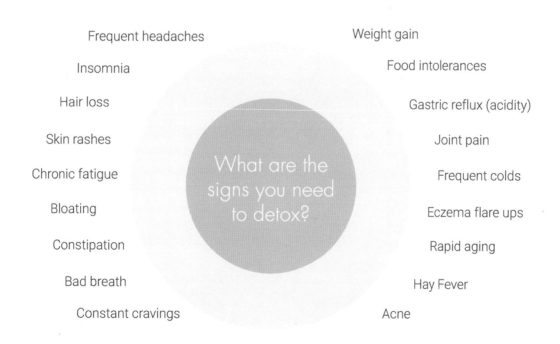

Frequent headaches

Weight gain

Insomnia

Food intolerances

Hair loss

Gastric reflux (acidity)

Skin rashes

Joint pain

Chronic fatigue

What are the signs you need to detox?

Frequent colds

Bloating

Eczema flare ups

Constipation

Rapid aging

Bad breath

Hay Fever

Constant cravings

Acne

# 1.2 BENEFITS OF DETOXING & FASTING

✔ Boost your immune system to fight against illness.

✔ Renew your energy and vitality to recharge your life with newfound vigor.

✔ Improve sleep and enjoy restorative and rejuvenating nights.

✔ Boost your metabolism to shed excess weight and feel lighter.

✔ Experience radiant skin and voluminous hair for a glowing appearance.

✔ Improve your mood and experience a more positive outlook.

✔ Boost your fertility and grow your family.

✔ Reduce your blood pressure and support your cardiovascular health.

✔ Slow down the aging process and experience a youthful look and feel.

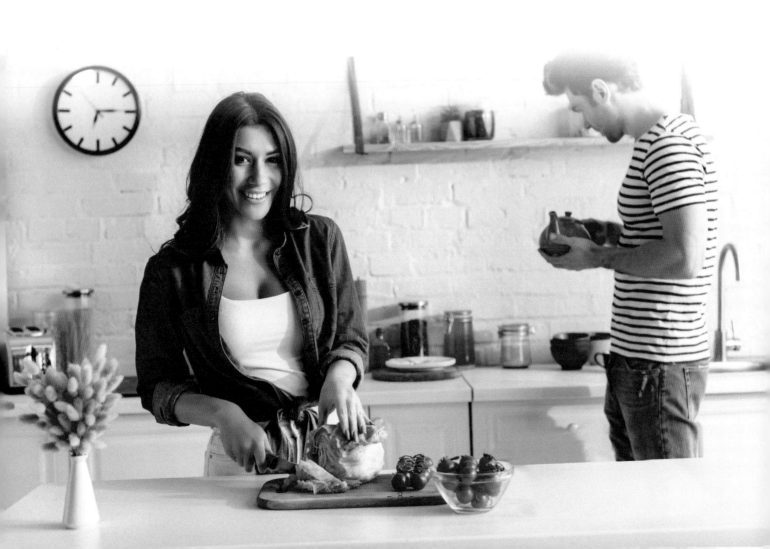

# II. THE SCIENCE

**Health begins in the gut** – the root system of the human body. According to the Austrian physician and researcher, Dr. F. X. Mayr (1875 – 1965), the chronic digestive damage, caused by toxicity overload, is what makes a person sick, prematurely old, and unattractive.

Scientific research on the role of the **microbiome and metabolome** is becoming more and more intensive currently. Claude Bernard (1813 to 1878), founder of modern physiology, first described "intestinal autointoxication" around 1870. This was further researched by Elia Metchnikoff (1845-1916), the founder of modern immunology. In 1908 he published his findings in his book "Prolongation of Life" and, based on this knowledge, F.X. Mayr (1875-1965) developed his concept for the treatment of "intestinal autointoxication", which is still highly effective today. [1]

The concept of **"silent inflammation"** has been recognized as the cause of chronic disease for some time already, but lately is increasingly being supplemented by the concept of **"silent intoxication"**.

Thus, the connections between the gut environment and body organs are being closely studied. It appears that organs first experience intoxication, followed by inflammation. The representation published in EMBO Report[2] is not complete. For example, there is also a Gut-Skin Axis, meaning a causal connection between the gut and skin diseases.

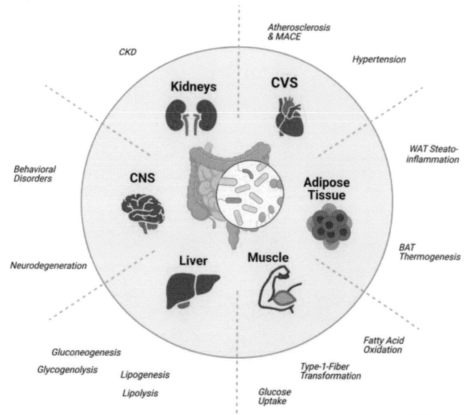

Source: EMBO Reports 2022 2, Vol 23 (10) Fig. 2
https://www.ncbi.nlm.nih.gov/pmc/articles/PMC9535759/pdf/EMBR-23-e55664.pdf

**What is new?** It is the differentiation in the evaluation of the milieu in the feces. The milieu depends on the selection of our food and the quality of chewing and digestion. Some of the putrefactive toxins produced intestinally are strongly alkaline[3]. If there is also a lack of lactic acid and short-chain fatty acids (SCFA) in the intestinal lumen, the result is a stool pH of well over 7. This is chronically common and detectable in most so-called "civilized" worlds. **Permanent adjustment of the stool pH to 6.0** (and first morning urine /saliva pH 7 – 8) **is an essential goal of the Upgraders® method.**

The pH value of the stool (environment in the intestinal lumen) is considered and evaluated differently from the pH of the urine and saliva (approximate statement about the pH in the body tissue). They are different compartments and organ systems. Since the measurement in the stool is unpleasant, we have limited ourselves here to the determination of the pH in the urine and saliva.

To determine pH levels, use Urine pH papers to test and record urine for the first morning pH (normal urine pH readings: 7 – 8). If the pH reading is lower than 7, alkalization and diet adjustment is recommended. During the time of alkalizing, urinary pH will generally test 7.4 and higher, which is desired for the biochemical reactions to shift the acid out of the tissues and body. Continue to alkalize until consistent readings are achieved in the normal pH range. This process can take months to balance the milieu and should be monitored with pH testing until the ideal range is obtained.

**The optimal health is possible only if bacterial toxins are eliminated and are not forming again.**[2, 4]

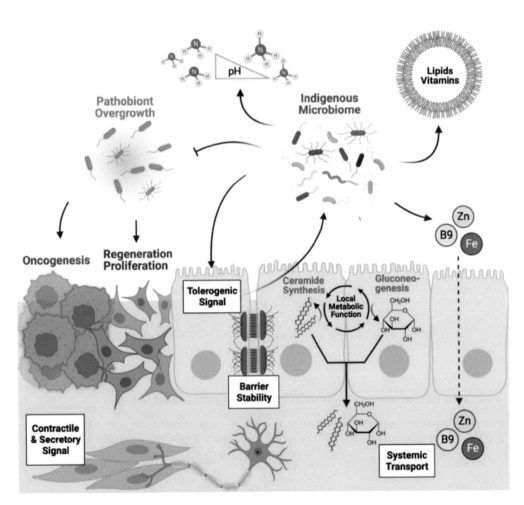

Source: EMBO Reports 2022, Vol 23 (10) Fig. 1
https://www.ncbi.nlm.nih.gov/pmc/articles/PMC9535759/pdf/EMBR-23-e55664.pdf

Studies show that even the slightest imbalance in the digestive system significantly limits muscular and neurological performance[5,6,7].

**What does an optimal health in the digestive system mean?**

---

**NUTRITION = FOOD x DIGESTION**

---

The function of the digestive system has to be restored before better nourishment of the organism can take place. **As long as the "digestion" is flawed, the body cannot be adequately nourished.**

**Right "food"** is the result of selection, quality, quantity and the cooking method. It requires:

- ✔ Balance within the macronutrients (carbohydrates, fats, proteins)
- ✔ Optimal supply of micronutrients (vital substances incl. biophotons, electrons and enzymes, minerals, trace elements)
- ✔ Fiber, herbs, and spices that regulate the intestinal environment
- ✔ Lowest possible levels of toxins and inhibitors (heavy metals, pesticides, hormones, antibiotics etc.)
- ✔ Optimal preparation of meals with emphasis on preservation of vital substances
- ✔ Optimal time management of meals throughout the day

One of the main causes of reduced performance of all organs is **incorrect digestion** (= dyspepsia = maldigestion) [8].

---

**100% NUTRITION (FOOD x DIGESTION) = 0% SILENT INTOXICATION**

---

**Good "Digestion"** means food eaten slowly, in a relaxed state. Food eaten hastily will lead to incomplete digestion and to the following chain reactions[7]:

- ✔ Increased diffusion pressure of the toxins into the enterocytes and the surrounding tissue, blood and lymph
- ✔ Shift of the microbiome (intestinal flora) towards fermentation and/or putrefaction or other decay processes (=dyspepsia)
- ✔ Toxic metabolites produced in the intestines (dyspepsia toxins) paralyze the intestinal muscles
- ✔ Slowed passage of the chyme in the small intestine or of the stool in the large intestine
- ✔ More time for the production of toxic metabolites
- ✔ More time for the reabsorption of water from the stool (stool hardening, constipation)
- ✔ Increase in the concentration of toxic metabolites (endogenous toxins) in the colon
- ✔ Silent auto-intoxication
- ✔ Damage to the intestinal wall cells, malabsorption, carbohydrate intolerance, leaky gut, immunological food intolerance or allergies
- ✔ Damage to muscles, nervous system, immune system, vascular system, skin, eyes etc. [7,9]
- ✔ Activation of the immune system and silent inflammation
- ✔ Reduced performance of all mitochondria, cells and organs
- ✔ Oncogenesis

# Silent Intoxication

Before the "silent inflammation" usually comes the "silent intoxication".

Many diet guidelines focus on increased protein and reduced levels of carbohydrates. **However, large amounts of protein can only be digested if there are enough digestive enzymes available.**

Putrefaction and putrefaction processes in the intestines are known to be caused by incomplete digestion of proteins. Even the smallest deficiencies of enzymes lead to incorrect digestion. **The most common cause of such enzyme deficits is the lack of saliva in the swallowed food.** The oral saliva does contain relevant amounts of proteases. If protein is not optimally chewed and salivated in the mouth, and if it is not sufficiently digested by the acid in the stomach (note: proton pump inhibitors, PPI), the result is an incomplete enzymatic breakdown of the proteins into amino acids. The number of proteases and peptidases available and produced may not be sufficient to cleave 100% of all flooding proteins. Most of the undigested residual proteins or peptides are then not reabsorbed, but further decomposed by the proteolytic bacteria (proteobacteria, H2S-formers, certain clostridia, etc.) in the intestine[10].

**This results in metabolites that have cytotoxic properties[11].**

The best known and best researched key player is ammonia.

### AMMONIA INDUCED MITOCHONDRIAL DYSFUNCTION

Evidence of the formation of ammonia and other putrefactive and decomposing toxins in the intestines came about 90 years ago[12]

These endogenous toxins (particularly putrefactive toxins) have been shown to damage the mitochondria in all cells of the body[13]. Our nerve cells are particularly sensitive to this, as they have about 10 times more mitochondria per cell than most other cells in the body. Current studies show the connection between e.g. ammonia from the intestine and an encephalopathy (brain disease), which usually first manifests itself in the sense of general exhaustion[13]. As the intoxication increases, the reduction (degeneration) of all functions of the central nervous system (CNS) takes place: burnout, forgetfulness, memory loss up to dementia[14,15,16], mood swings up to depression, Parkinson's disease etc.

End products of intestinal putrefaction are: **ammonia, skatole, p-cresol, TMA/TMAO, LPS, indoxyl-sulfate, phenols, cadaverine, …. Most of those substances are dose-dependently toxic and carcinogenic** [17].

The environment in the intestinal lumen (small and large intestine) determines whether the bacteria produce either toxic or protective metabolites.[18]

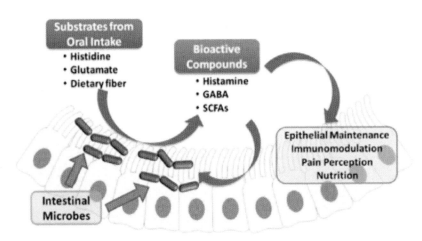

Source: Hemarajata, P. and Versalovic, J: Ther Adv Gastroenterol (2013) 6(1) 39-51

In this context, "hepatic encephalopathy" has best been scientifically researched. Ammonia plays the major role in its pathogenesis [12,19].

## TMA / TMAO

Another group of substances has been increasingly researched in recent years: TMA (trimethyl-amine), the substance that gives rotting fish its smell, and TMAO (trimethylamine-N-oxide). Recent research focuses on cardiovascular risk [20].

However, like ammonia, TMA is a putrefactive toxin produced in the gut by proteolytic bacteria. TMA is converted to TMAO in the liver.

**This toxin (TMA) also reduces mitochondrial function[20, 21, 22].**

**The pH in the stool is a decisive regulator**

In the context of Alzheimer's research, it was noticed that certain bile acids are produced in the intestine and damage the brain after reabsorption[15,23].

In particular, ursodeoxycholic acid (UDCA), "unique secondary bile acids (Bas), such as iso-3-oxo-, allo-, 3-oxoallo-, and isoallo-lithocholic acid (LCA)" are considered to be protective against silent inflammation [24].

Cytotoxic bile acids (e.g., deoxycholic acid, DCA) are produced when stool pH rises above 6.5. The enzymes that decide whether neuroprotective or cytotoxic bile acids are produced are (like almost all enzymes) pH-sensitive.

> **The higher the pH in the stool, the more cytotoxic and the less neuroprotective bile acids are produced.**

The relevance of these findings was recently discussed and confirmed in a Nature publication by Sato et al. from 07/29/2021 on microbiome research on centenarians [24].

**Other toxic metabolites from the gut include:** Quinolinic acid (from tryptophan), hippuric acid, HPHPA (3-(3-hydroxyphenyl)-3-hydroxypropionic acid), indoxyl sulfate, p-cresol sulfate, phenylacetylglutamine, tryptamine (depends on the level produced) ...

These have become detectable and measurable in daily practice with unprecedented precision in special laboratories such as BIOVIS. Only ammonia is so unstable that it breaks down on the way to the laboratory and is not detectable in the stool.

**Effect of metabolites on stool pH**

On the one hand, all of these metabolites have a more or less strong, molecule-specific influence on the ambient pH. On the other hand, the total pH of the stool is also related to the amount of fermenting and glandular acids (such as gastric and bile acids). Ammonia is the most important base. Lactic and butyric acid are the most relevant acids. The gastric acid is neutralized by the bicarbonate of the pancreatic juice in the upper small intestine, taking it from a pH of approx. 1.5 to a pH between 4.0 to 4.5, and therefore plays a subordinate role for the stool pH. Only in the case of gastric acid weakness (e.g. in atrophic gastritis) does the lack of gastric acid have a double negative effect: as a lack of acid itself and via the lack of denaturation (see below) as a promoter of putrefaction dyspepsia.

**Acidifying flora protects against putrefactive toxins**

At the beginning of the 20th century, Ilja Iljitsch Metschnikow described Lactobacillus bulgaricus and its correlation with longevity and the health span. **The lactic acid of the acidifying flora became an anti-aging agent.**

Actinobacteria and Proteobacteria compete for food in the gut. They try to poison each other. The **Actinobacteria (healthy acidification flora)** form e.g. **lactate and butyrate** in order to prevent the proteobacteria from growing via an acidic environment. The latter need it alkaline. Conversely, in an alkaline milieu, **Proteobacteria produce putrefaction toxins, which act as inhibitors for the acidification flora[25,26].**

Actinobacteria mainly metabolize carbohydrates, simple sugars, oligosaccharides, starch, but also pectins, glucans and fructans - i.e. prebiotic roughage from vegetables, herbs and cereals.

**If you want to increase the number of Actinobacteria and their metabolic activity, you should refrain from insulinogenic sugars, add prebiotic fiber and promote the acidic environment in the intestine. The acidification flora can also be favorably influenced by milieu-stabilizing probiotics.**

The so-called "cross-feeding" takes place between bifidobacteria and lactobacilli forming D-lactate and the butyrate-formers further processing the D-lactate into short-chain fatty acids.

**So, if you feed the lactate-formers and also add the dextrorotatory lactic acid via fermented vegetables or their juice, Kefir and soured milk products to the food you create ideal conditions for homeostasis in the gut.**

**Strong energy-forming and anti-inflammatory abilities have been proven especially for the Faecalibacterium Prausnitzii and the butyrate builders.**

- Butyric acid can protect against chronic inflammatory bowel disease (IBD) and colon cancer.
- Patients with Crohn's disease are also deficient in Faecalibacterium prausnitzii, a butyrate-forming bacterium that secretes substances that have anti-inflammatory effects on gut cells by blocking NF-κB activation and IL-8 production[27] .

**At what point is fermentation pathological?**

Today, fermentation in the gut is only considered pathological as the cause of disease if the pH in the stool falls well below 5.5.

The consistency of the stool then usually takes on a liquid consistency and smells very sour. This is a rather rare occurrence today compared to the frequency of slow transit constipation.

The therapeutic approach here would be to dramatically reduce the intake of carbohydrates - especially sugar - but without reducing the resistant starch = complex, cross-linked carbohydrates, roughage(!). **Fasting or eating a "ketogenic diet = carbohydrate fasting" then leads to a new flora balance** and stops the supply of substrate for the putrefaction dyspepsia.

### Slow Transit Constipation

Most people in the so-called "**Western way of life**" show a "**slow transit constipation**" **with a firm consistency and a stool pH of 7 to 9**, rarely even higher, due to the serious lack of dietary fiber. Because this putrefaction weakens the mitochondria of the gut wall, F.X. Mayr correctly described the "weak small intestine" as a far underestimated problem of mankind, about 100 years ago, already.

### Food Intolerances

According to Bodo Kuklinski, most food intolerances are caused by exactly that: weakened enterocytes [28]. He writes: "**Lactose, gluten and fructose intolerance are given as causes of unclear abdominal symptoms. These are consequences of mitochondrial cytopathy with secondary vitamin B12 deficiency.**" (Author's note: ... because B12 in the terminal ileum can only be actively reabsorbed in vital, ATP-filled enterocytes.)

### Flashback to the Stone Age

During the longest period of human existence, 10 times more fiber from leaves and roots was eaten than nowadays. This formerly led to the profuse formation of Firmicutes and Actinobacteria. Solid stools with a pH above 6.5 were extremely rare in those times. The normal stool consistency of mankind before the beginning of the agricultural age (10,000 years ago) was that of a cow pat in "normal transit".

### Diversity

The diversity of the flora-bacteria (microbiota) in the intestine has been correlated in many scientific works with the overall health of humans in various respects.

> Great diversity in the microbiota is achieved
> through great diversity in food.

The types of vegetables, herbs and spices are particularly important here. A meal should contain more than 30 different fragments of it, e.g. all the colors of nature.

With this background knowledge, the recommendation to avoid foods in case of intolerances must be re-evaluated. Under no circumstances should the recommendation to avoid eating what you do not tolerate during a certain time lead to a long-term monotonous diet with limited diversity. Food that is combined in a variety of ways and eaten slowly reduces the tendency to react with signs of food intolerance as the vitality of the intestines increases under those circumstances.

**Conclusions:**

Vegetables that have been pre-digested enzymatically (fermented) before being eaten and which, **without pasteurization**, bring along living fermentation bacteria as well as the ferments (enzymes) and the end products, the acids, are an ideal support for the healthy acid environment. These vegetables are not raw, precisely because they are pre-digested, yet they have not - and should not have- been heated.

**As the amount of fermented vegetables eaten per day increases, the pH in the stool decreases. The consistency of the stool becomes softer as the portions of fermented vegetables increase.**

"Sauerkraut is the body's chimney sweep" as the saying goes.

### Histamine

If you talk about sauerkraut, the immediate objection is that there is incompatibility because of the histamine it contains. This objection is obsolete as shown by the following considerations:

Fermented foods naturally contain certain amounts of histamine, depending on how ripe they are. Histamine is formed during the enzymatic breakdown of the amino acid histidine, which 'in turn' is a component of most proteins. With a high-protein diet and poor digestion (putrefaction dyspepsia), most people already have high histamine levels.

Ammonia, as a putrefactive toxin, blocks the diamine oxidase DAO and thus the breakdown of histamine.

> Histamine intolerance is a putrefactive disease!
> The less putrefaction, the less histamine intolerance!

Therefore, **after Upgraders® 21-day Health & Beauty Pro Detox & Intermittent Fasting program, the DAO as well as the histamine-degrading histamine-N-methyltransferases (HNMTs) work better again.** This is the ideal time to stimulate the epigenetics to produce DAO and histamine-N-methyltransferases (HNMTs). If there was not too much putrefaction in the intestines, in most cases this has been regulated down by just avoiding foods containing histamine.

As with muscle training, the degradation capacity is increased with a (carefully) increasing dose of histamine. Ultimately, such histamine intolerance is treated curatively. The permanent avoidance of histamine is therefore not a solution to the problem.

The only exceptions are people with rare, genetically determined DAO polymorphisms or severe IgE allergies. However, the latter still benefit in the long run from a correction of the intestinal balance according to the criteria described here.

**Diagnostics of maldigestion**

Clinical setting:

- ✔ Manual examination of the abdomen is highly recommended - there should be no palpable resistance, but a normal bowel tone under the abdominal wall.
- ✔ No sensitivity to pressure (especially in the area of the ileocaecal transition and the root of mesentery)
- ✔ No congestion in the area of the descending colon and sigmoid colon
- ✔ No significant accumulation of gas in the colon and certainly not in the small intestine (SIBO)
- ✔ Tongue without furrows, coating and edge impressions
- ✔ Skin without acne, eczema and edema
- ✔ Posture of the spine without protective reactions (especially of the iliopsoas muscle on both sides)
- ✔ Stool frequency 1-2 per day without pressing
- ✔ Smooth and soft sausage-shaped or blobs-shaped stool (Bristol Stool Scale type 4-5) with rounded ends and a smooth surface. It sinks in water because it has no gaseous impurities and has only a slight characteristic odor. A healthy intestine evacuates the stool cleanly, which is why any noticeable soiling of the anal region is an indication of damage to the intestinal tract.

Laboratory technology:

- ✔ pH in the stool: 6.0 (± 0.2) is a must!
- ✔ Water content 82 to 88%
- ✔ Fecal calprotectin <17.9 mg/l
- ✔ Fecal alpha 1-antitrypsin <10 mg/dl
- ✔ Fecal zonulin <30 ng/ml
- ✔ Diversity of the intestinal flora >6
- ✔ Ratio Actinobacteria / Proteobacteria >2
- ✔ Optimum numbers and function of the acidifying flora, especially the butyrate formers
- ✔ Sum of straight-chain fatty acids in the stool > 250 mmol/l with a high proportion of butyrate
- ✔ No putrefactive toxins detectable

According to current research results, the special microbiome and metabolome as well as digestive marker analysis mentioned above is suitable for detecting incorrect digestion.

As already mentioned, some of the putrefactive toxins influence the pH value in the stool in the direction of a pH increase (alkaline). A lack of acidifying flora also increases the pH of the stool.

Therefore, measuring the pH value in the stool is both inexpensive and efficient and therefore very useful for follow-up controls.

The usual litmus paper strip, which is otherwise used for determining the urine pH, is also useful for this purpose.

> The optimal pH in the stool is 6.0.

## Conclusion

The fastest and most thorough therapy for putrefaction dyspepsia (without consulting a specialized doctor) is the **Upgraders® 21-day Health & Beauty Pro Detox & Intermittent Fasting program**.

- ✔ Eliminating or avoiding any maldigestion is the primary focus of the Upgraders® Method. Optimal abdominal balance is always a "conditio sine qua non".

- ✔ According to the current state of research, the relationship between fermentation and putrefaction in the intestine must be reassessed.

- ✔ A permanently stable state of health of the intestines and thus of the entire organism can only be achieved with optimal support of the acidifying flora with the aim of: pH 6.0 in the stool.

- ✔ The best possible promotion of the acidifying flora requires fermented foods in an individually appropriate dose and variety.

> **It is our primary target to reach a stool pH of 6.0 (or first morning saliva pH 7 – 8) in 21 days with the Upgraders® 21-day Health & Beauty Pro Detox & Intermittent Fasting program.**

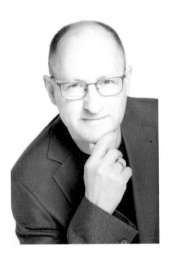

Vienna, Austria January 2024

Dr. med. Henning Sartor

# III. What is UPGRADERS® Method

## 3.1 A BALANCING ACT: THE GUIDE TO UPGRADERS® METHOD

## OPTIMAL HEALTH THROUGH A CLEAN LIFE BLUEPRINT

**Master Daily Detoxification: Heal, Lose Weight, Sleep Better, Look Younger, and Thrive.**

True health starts with eliminating gut toxins that affect nutrient uptake. Cleansing at the cellular level corrects gut and metabolic balance, boosting the body's own healing abilities. This process enhances overall health, improves appearance, boosts energy, and sharpens mental clarity.

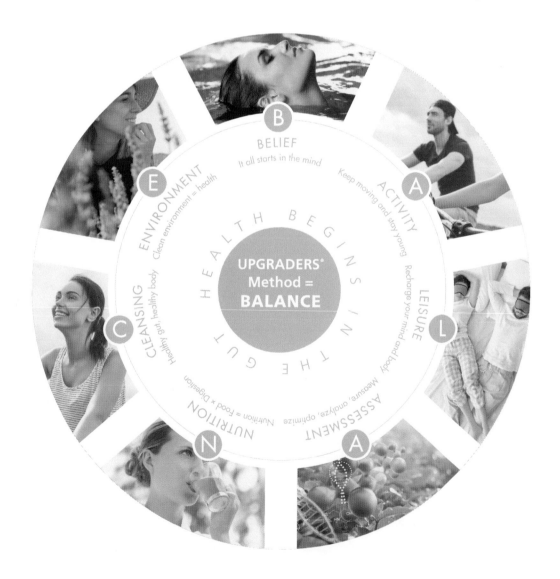

Start your journey to upgraded health and beauty today by taking the Toxicity Quiz at upgraders.com!

# 3.2 OUR EDGE:
# HOW UPGRADERS® METHOD WORKS

**Experience the Upgraders® Method: a 21-day, clinic-grade home detox program. It rejuvenates your cells through a lifestyle program, powered by potent, all-natural supplements, made from bioactive ingredients. Targeting toxin overload, it helps you heal, lose weight, sleep better, look younger and thrive.**

Our groundbreaking cellular cleanse meticulously restores your body's natural nutrient and acid-base balance, unlocking the pinnacle of nutrient absorption for revitalization and renewal. A detoxified body maximizes nutrient intake, fostering health, weight loss, improved sleep, and timeless anti-aging benefits. The detox and fasting strategically eliminate bacterial toxins and address silent inflammation—a root cause of many chronic health issues.

Our 21-day program isn't just a cleanse; it's a holistic metabolic re-balancing solution.

*Our 21-Day DIY Detox and Intermittent Fasting Program draws inspiration from the renowned Austrian physician Dr. Franz Xaver Mayr (1875-1965) and his century-old clinic detox – a trusted therapeutic approach still employed by exclusive European wellness clinics today. Rediscover centuries-old wisdom, now within reach.*

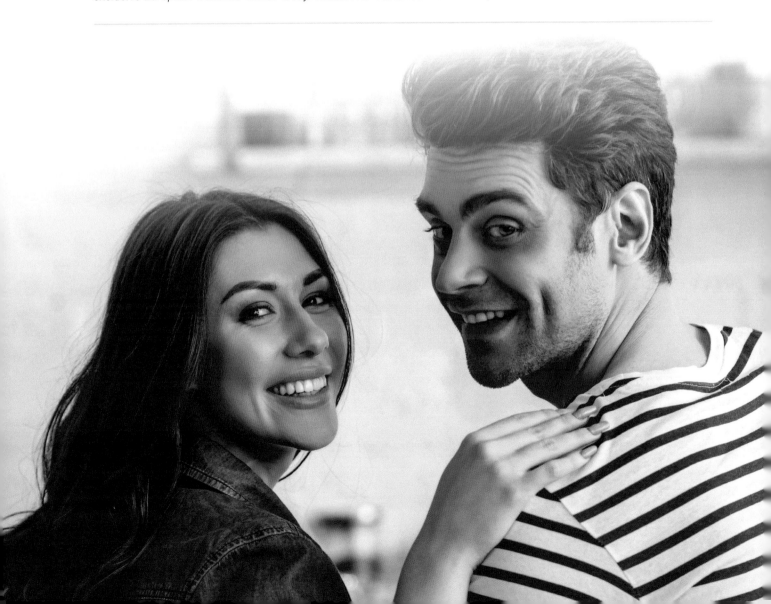

# 21 DAYS TO MAXIMUM NOURISHMENT: A KEY TO UPGRADED HEALTH & BEAUTY

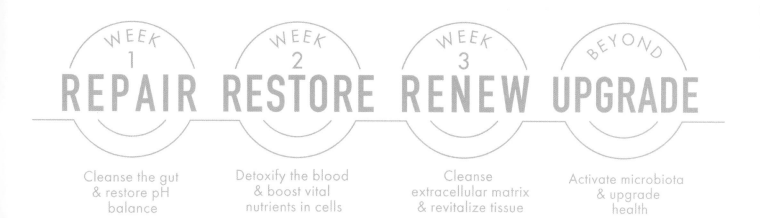

WEEK 1
REPAIR
Cleanse the gut & restore pH balance

WEEK 2
RESTORE
Detoxify the blood & boost vital nutrients in cells

WEEK 3
RENEW
Cleanse extracellular matrix & revitalize tissue

BEYOND
UPGRADE
Activate microbiota & upgrade health

The 21-day period aligns with the body's regeneration cycle, promoting deep cellular detoxification. **Begin feeling and looking better already after the first 7 days!**

Explore solutions at upgraders.com.

# 3.3 THE POWER OF SUPPLEMENTS – OVERCOMING MALNUTRITION

To conceptualize the relationship between malnutrition, its causes and interventions:

## MALNUTRITION = POOR DIETARY CHOICES x INEFFICIENT DIGESTION
⤷ Toxin Buildup ⟶ 'Silent' Inflammation

• **POOR DIETARY CHOICES** should be addressed by enhancing the diet with nutritious foods and appropriate supplementation.

• **INEFFICIENT DIGESTION** necessitates support through bowel cleansing and detoxification to promote better nutrient absorption and reduce toxicity.

---

Intestinal rehabilitation through **UPGRADERS® supplements**, or microbiome re-balancing, targets four key gut health objectives:

## 1. CLEANSE
This step involves minimizing or eliminating elements detrimental to beneficial microorganisms. Key practices include reducing stress, avoiding chemicals and pharmaceuticals (notably antibiotics), cutting out smoking, sugar, white flour, all gluten and limiting alcohol ideally to none. DETOXIFICATION is a critical component of this phase, exemplified by the **UPGRADERS® 21-day Health & Beauty Pro Detox & Intermittent Fasting program and its set of tools for success.** When detoxing or fasting, it is vital to provide your body with antioxidants, phytonutrients, essential fats, B-vitamins, enzymes, prebiotics, and probiotics. These are the essential tools your organs need for effective cleansing and metabolic rebalancing. **Our expertly formulated supplement program is tailor-made to boost and strengthen your body's natural detoxification processes.**

**REMOVING TOXINS AT A CELLULAR LEVEL ENHANCES SUPPLEMENTS' EFFECTIVENESS, ENSURING MAXIMUM NUTRIENT ABSORPTION FOR OPTIMAL NOURISHMENT.**

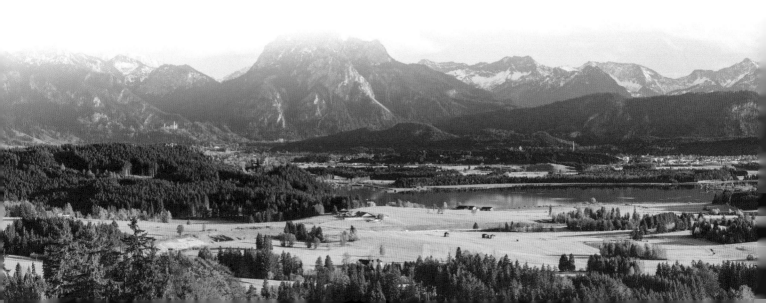

## 2. PROBIOTICS

Our supplements introduce **essential living microorganisms** to support gut flora, promoting gut health and function with precise bacterial strains e.g. lactate and butyrate.

**Fermented foods** such as sauerkraut, kimchi, and kefir are packed with probiotics that boost gut health by nourishing good bacteria and reducing cravings. These beneficial probiotics help maintain a healthy digestive system, crucial for your overall well-being.

## 3. PREBIOTICS

**Essential dietary fibers** like cellulose, found abundantly in high-fiber foods such as lettuce, vegetables, and whole grains, nourish and sustain beneficial microorganisms, fostering a flourishing microbiome. The difference between feeling bloated and not can often be attributed to fiber consumption.

## 4. MULTIVITAMINS & MINERALS

By supplementing with **essential micronutrients**, you provide crucial support to metabolic and enzymatic systems.  People in the northern hemisphere should add **vitamin D** supplements to their routine during the darker months to support bone health and immune function. It is also important to supplement **Omega 3** in order to build up proper membranes and prevent cardiovascular disease i.e Olive oil (containing Omega 6 & 3) or Linseed (or flaxseed) oil, which is anti-inflammatory (containing mainly ALA) or pure Omega 3 oils from fish or vegan from seaweed (containing mainly EPA and DHA).

Despite the abundance of vitamins, overeating and lavish diets can still impair their benefits, leading to a decline in health. Remember, too much of anything, including raw foods, can be harmful.

Nowadays, our bodies struggle to get sufficient minerals and trace elements, a problem exacerbated by environmental pollution and the resulting demineralization of plants, our primary food sources. Our fast-paced lifestyles further amplify our need for **essential minerals such as potassium, magnesium, and calcium**. To address these deficiencies, modern therapies recommend boosting intake of these minerals, particularly to neutralize stress. By the way, the consumption of alcohol, coffee and various medications, as well as excessive intake of sugar, fruits and heavy grains, can lead to a depletion of our mineral reserves. These "mineral robbers" not only disrupt our digestive system but also contribute to over-acidification, negatively affecting our metabolism. The UPGRADERS® Method seeks to mitigate these issues by lowering body acidity, showcasing its role as an effective therapeutic strategy.

Each of these four steps is designed to work synergistically, creating a balanced and healthy gut ecosystem, pivotal for overall well-being, and vitality.

Explore solutions at upgraders.com.

CLEAN LIFE
UPGRADERS®
CERTIFIED

# CHOOSING NATURAL OVER SYNTHETIC

Our **'Clean Living' certification** reflects our dedication to unwavering excellence and the highest quality standards. Begin a transformative health journey with **UPGRADERS® supplements**, meticulously developed by world-renowned medical experts and naturopaths, designed to harness the full potential of natural nutrients.

Immerse yourself in the strength of 100% natural, non-toxic, and bioactive formulations, thoughtfully packaged in eco-friendly, biodegradable materials. Our commitment to excellence is rooted in the understanding that plant-based, **all-natural supplements, enriched with plant co-factors, ensure superior bioavailability compared to synthetic alternatives**.

## 'CLEAN LIFE CERTIFIED' QUALITY STANDARDS

**100% NATURAL**
Harnessing Nature's Power: Certified plant formulas infused with natural, active ingredients for maximum effectiveness.

**TOXIN FREE**
100% Clean: Additive-free, chemical-free, quality-certified ingredients and products (ISO, GMP, HACCP).

**EFFECTIVE**
Unparalleled Potency: : Our bioactive ingredients are meticulously sourced, lab-tested and highly concentrated.

**HEALTH BEGINS IN THE GUT ...**
The gut microbiota and the immune system work together to impact organ functions through connections such as gut–brain, gut–skin, gut–bone and beyond.

**SUSTAINABLE**
Green & Clean: Our eco-conscious products use natural ingredients and responsible practices for a sustainable, toxin-free choice.

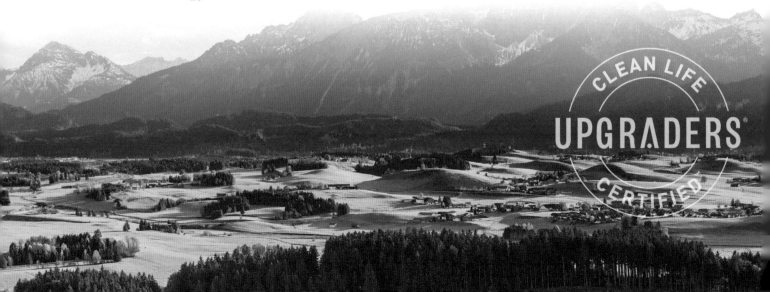

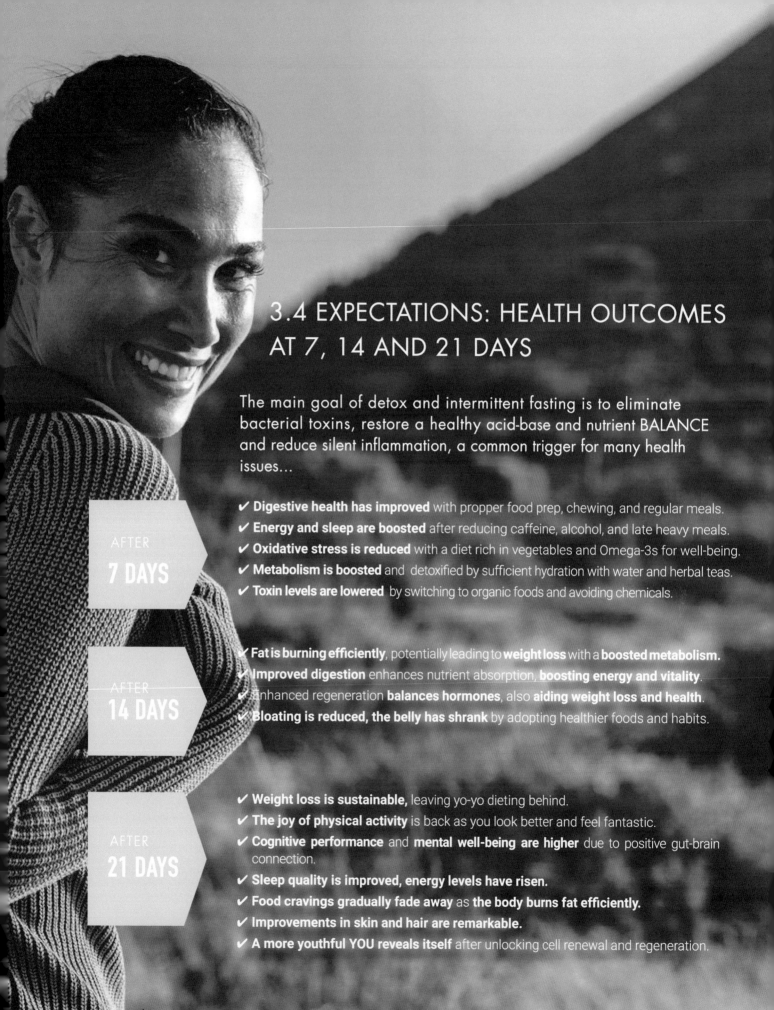

# 3.4 EXPECTATIONS: HEALTH OUTCOMES AT 7, 14 AND 21 DAYS

The main goal of detox and intermittent fasting is to eliminate bacterial toxins, restore a healthy acid-base and nutrient BALANCE and reduce silent inflammation, a common trigger for many health issues...

**AFTER 7 DAYS**

✔ **Digestive health has improved** with propper food prep, chewing, and regular meals.
✔ **Energy and sleep are boosted** after reducing caffeine, alcohol, and late heavy meals.
✔ **Oxidative stress is reduced** with a diet rich in vegetables and Omega-3s for well-being.
✔ **Metabolism is boosted** and detoxified by sufficient hydration with water and herbal teas.
✔ **Toxin levels are lowered** by switching to organic foods and avoiding chemicals.

**AFTER 14 DAYS**

✔ **Fat is burning efficiently**, potentially leading to **weight loss** with a **boosted metabolism**.
✔ **Improved digestion** enhances nutrient absorption, **boosting energy and vitality**.
✔ Enhanced regeneration **balances hormones**, also **aiding weight loss and health**.
✔ **Bloating is reduced, the belly has shrank** by adopting healthier foods and habits.

**AFTER 21 DAYS**

✔ **Weight loss is sustainable,** leaving yo-yo dieting behind.
✔ **The joy of physical activity** is back as you look better and feel fantastic.
✔ **Cognitive performance** and **mental well-being are higher** due to positive gut-brain connection.
✔ **Sleep quality is improved, energy levels have risen.**
✔ **Food cravings gradually fade away** as **the body burns fat efficiently.**
✔ **Improvements in skin and hair are remarkable.**
✔ **A more youthful YOU reveals itself** after unlocking cell renewal and regeneration.

# 3.5 STORIES OF HEALTH TRANSFORMATIONS

" No spin, no waffle, no sales or gimmick... just follow the instructions and everything will work exactly the way it is meant to do. This is a very well-thought-out kit, a few of these things that come on the market are spin but this is the top-of-the-market stuff. The guide is good, there is plenty of instruction but also detailed information. I am sleeping like a log and I am very aware that my body has cleansed itself. My energy levels are through the roof and that is the best bit, it took about 4 days for the lethargy to leave me but once it was gone I began to notice such a bounce and such clarity of thinking after day 8. A great detox, a journey to be done with joy, try to keep positive about the difficult days, you are going to be giving your body a gift... a real gift to be cherished.

- Amazon customer, UK

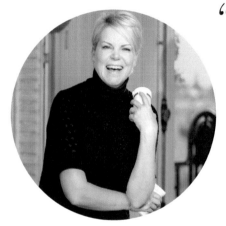

" As I am 52 and going through menopause I felt more clear headed and stronger as well. Upgraders 3 week cleanse was life changing for me! I have always struggled with consistent constipation and had developed bad eating habits that had led to weight gain and bloating. Starting on the program the first 5 days were intense, as my system started to detox and release things that had been trapped for years. By day 6 my headaches had disappeared and my skin was clear and my energy levels were amazing. My system was flushing at a regular pace and as the days progressed I simply felt better that I can ever remember! As I am 52 and going through menopause I felt more clear headed and stronger as well. Such a wonderful program and one I will begin to do regularly 1-2 times per year! Thank goodness someone finally developed a program like this that you can do at home and achieve these results. My weight is coming down at a healthy pace (I lost 4kg / ~9 pounds in 21 days) and even after I have finished I continue to stick to the dietary recommendations because I feel so good. I highly recommend this 3-week cleanse!!"

- JENNIFER V, 52 (France)

" The secret formula of staying young! Ever since I turned 50, I feel like my body is no longer the same. The answer from my doctors is that it's a hormone problem. Until I tried Upgraders 21-day program. I learned how our unhealthy lifestyle is responsible for high toxicity levels in our body driving inflammation / inflammaging. Once you fix the root cause, you fix everything. I gave it a try and the results were astonishing. Not only did I lose excess weight (4.5kg + it continues to come down slowly), I also started to sleep better, and have more energy to do more. My blood pressure has normalized which has not happened in the last 10 years. I will definitely do this program again after 6 months! This truly might be the secret of staying young :) "

- ANNA, 50 (UK)

❝ *I got pregnant right after the 21-day program! I suffered from few health issues like insomnia, fatigue, frequent colds so it looked like I need to do something to boost my immunity. I signed up with Upgraders 21-day program. The program is very easy and very clearly structured. All products have very high quality which you can feel during the programm. Every day I felt better and better. Amazing how 21 days can make a big difference to your health, energy levels, sleep, weight... And surprise, surprise, I got pregnant right after the 21-day program!!!! Thank you Upgraders for everything you do!"*

– SIMONE, 42 (Austria)

❝ *Clarity, energy, strength & beauty just after 1 week! The impact of this 21-day detox program has been truly remarkable. As a busy mother and someone who has battled the effects of Covid, I had been dealing with chronic fatigue, exhaustion, and insomnia. That's why I decided to give this program a try, as I had heard that toxins are at the root of the chaos within our bodies. The first few days were challenging as I could feel my body undergoing a transformation. However, on day 7, it was like a rebirth for me. I emerged with newfound clarity, energy, strength, and a beauty that I hadn't experienced in a long time. This detox program has become an essential part of my seasonal routine. I'm incredibly grateful for the positive changes it has brought into my life. Thank you!!!!"*

- MARTHA S. (Germany)

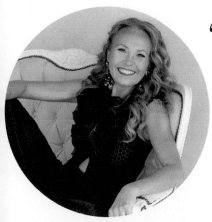

❝ *After completing the Upgraders program, I experienced a remarkable transformation. Each morning, I felt an incredible surge of energy that had been absent before, and friends and acquaintances began commenting on how I appeared better than ever. Over the three-week period, I also achieved a significant weight loss, shedding 4 kilograms. However, the most profound outcome for me was the newfound awareness and attention I developed towards my body and health. The Upgraders program not only delivered tangible results but also instilled in me a lasting commitment to prioritize my well-being. It has become a transformative journey that extends far beyond the initial three weeks, influencing my daily habits and fostering a positive impact on my overall health. I am deeply grateful for the Upgraders experience and the positive changes it has brought into my life."*

- ENE P. (Estonia)

## PROMOTE WELLNESS!

Now that you've experienced the incredible benefits of detox, why not share your journey with family, friends and co-workers?

**When you become an Affiliate Partner, your friends will enjoy an exclusive 11% discount on all their orders and you'll receive a generous 10% commission.**

Visit our 'Become a Partner' page on upgraders.com to discover more about our Affiliate program.

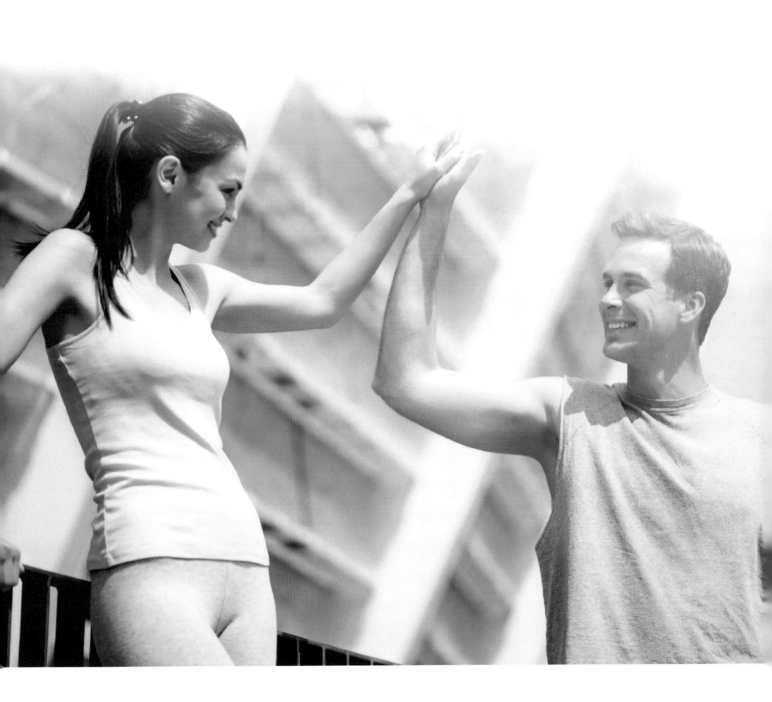

# IV. GETTING STARTED

## 4.1 SUCCESS BLUEPRINT: PLANNING FOR SUCCESS

### CHOOSE A QUIET TIME

- Start during a low-stress week to enhance detox effectiveness.
- Start Friday for ease.

### EXPECT EARLY SYMPTOMS

- Expect headaches, fatigue. Start reducing caffeine a week before to lessen headaches.
- 3L of spring water daily speeds up toxin removal.

### ESSENTIAL LIFESTYLE ADJUSTMENTS

- B = BELIEF: Incorporate mindfulness techniques i.e. meditation for stress relief.

- A = ACTIVITY: Walk and add gentle exercises like yoga.

- L = LEISURE: Ensure plenty of sleep and nap to aid recovery.

- A = ASSESSMENT: Assess your detox progress weekly.

- N = NUTRITION: Opt for fresh, organic foods, avoiding processed items.

- C = CLEANSING: Take UPGRADERS® supplements for cleanse and regeneration at cellular level.

- E = ENVIRONMENT: Minimize toxins in your surroundings and avoid energy-draining influences.

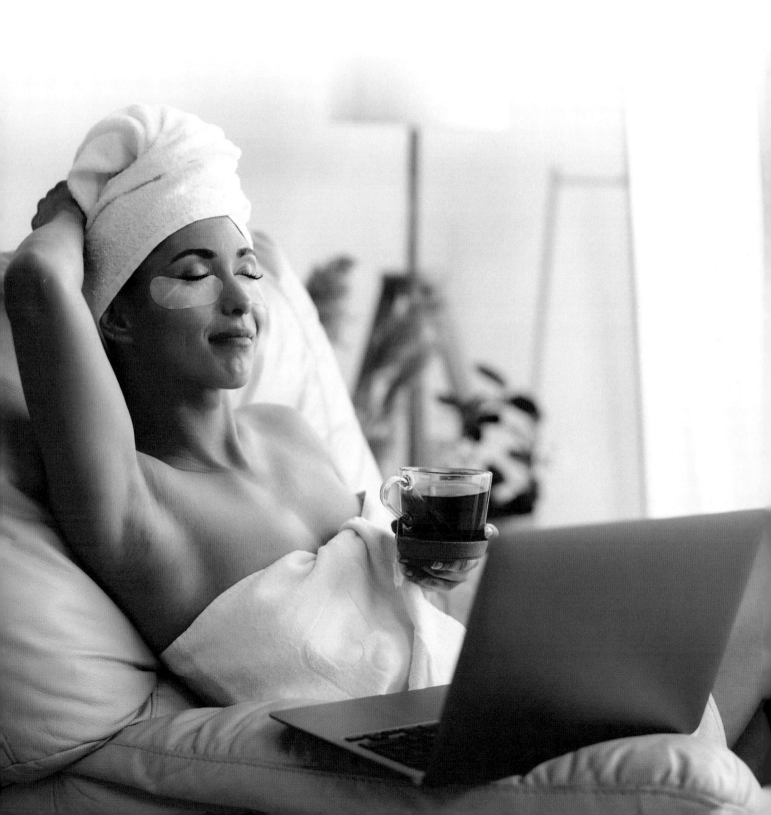

# 4.2 DETOX SUPPORT: MAXIMIZING YOUR DETOX EXPERIENCE

## DRY SKIN BRUSHING

Dry skin brushing is a vital practice for detoxification, helping to improve lymph and blood circulation while reducing cellulite. Begin each morning at your feet and brush upwards toward your heart, repeating the process for your arms, abdomen, and chest. Afterward, take a refreshing shower and apply a herbal detox massage oil (i.e. jojoba) to reduce puffiness and fluid retention.

## COLD THERAPIES

Alternating hot and cold showers (or only on legs and arms) invigorates your body, stimulates circulation, and aids in detoxification. This practice can boost your immune system, improve mood, and increase alertness, promoting overall well-being. Cryotherapy offers additional anti-inflammatory benefits.

## MASSAGES & COLONIC HYDROTHERAPIES

If you have access to massages and colonic hydrotherapies, consider incorporating them into your detox routine. A 60-minute lymphatic-drainage massage, a clinically proven detox technique, can be essential. It enhances blood flow, accelerate the elimination of excess lymph fluid, toxins, and fatty acids, ultimately reducing cellulite, bloating, and water retention. In addition, colonic hydrotherapies take your detox experience to the next level by addressing 400 reflex points during internal hydromassage, leaving you feel cleaned and revitalized.

## SAUNAS & INFRARED LIGHT CABIN

Saunas facilitate excretion of toxins through sweat via the largest organ of the body : the skin. Also experience the healing power of red light therapy, stimulating blood flow, catalysing natural cellular processes to relax muscles, fighting aging and rejuvenating the whole body.

## DETOX BATHS

Indulge in this soothing self-care ritual to unwind and rejuvenate. Enhance your relaxation by adding Epsom salt to a warm (not hot) bath for an amplified detox experience. Use this calming practice as needed to de-stress and promote your well-being. Alternatively, you can just soak your feet in an alkaline bath for 20 minutes.

## LIVER WRAP

Put a warm, damp towel (not over 40°C) on your stomach with a warm water bottle on top (on the right side) to aid liver function. Be cautious to avoid skin burns.

## WALKING

The average person naturally takes 3,000 to 6,000 daily steps during activities like commuting and shopping. Adding 30-40 minutes of walking (3,000 - 4,000 steps) helps meet the recommended 7,000 to 10,000 daily steps. Walking indirectly supports detox processes, enhances overall well-being, and crucially boosts oxygen supply for metabolism, along with improving blood flow, digestion, and stress reduction.

# V. UPGRADERS METHOD = BALANCE

 5.1 BELIEF: MINDFULNESS MAGIC

It all begins with the mind. Practicing mindfulness can enhance positive feelings, known as the optimism effect.

*"Our life is the creation of our mind."*
— *Buddha*

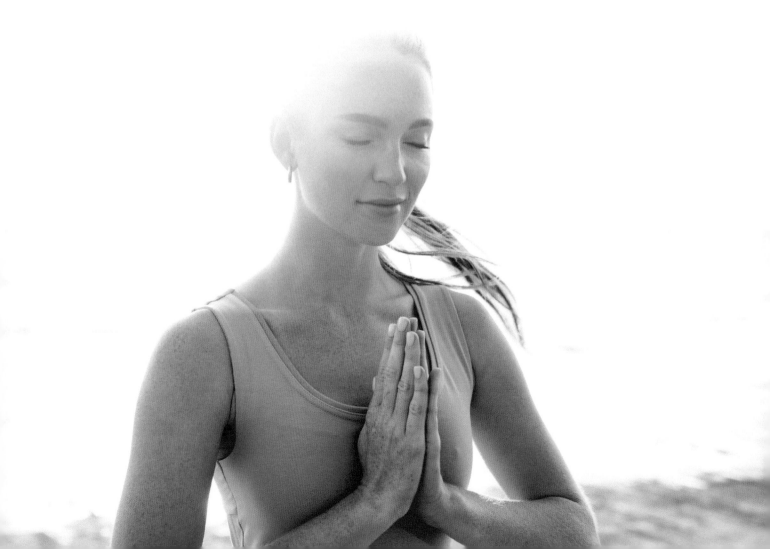

Scientific studies indicate that mindfulness may alleviate anxiety and depression, boost the immune system, aid in pain management, help break unhealthy habits, address insomnia, lower high blood pressure and positively impact the structure and function of the brain.

Mindfulness, described as the fundamental human ability to be fully present and aware of our surroundings, enables us to navigate through life without being overly reactive or overwhelmed. Many people turn to meditation for reasons such as stress reduction, anxiety management, sleep improvement and enhancement of emotional health, reflecting the broader impact of this practice on overall wellness [29, 30, 31, 32]. Meditation involves centering ourselves and spending waking time with brainwave frequencies in the 7-to-14 Hz range (the same frequency as dreaming during the REM sleep cycle). It entails focusing thoughts in a targeted manner with assistance from the subconscious. In this frequency, we solve problems, process conflicts and generate ideas.

**Transcendental meditation (TM)** stands out as the most effective and scientifically proven method for achieving meditative benefits. Here's a simple example of a meditation session:

| 1. PREPARATION: | 2. INTRODUCTION: | 3. MANTRAS: | 4. MAINTAIN FOCUS: | 5.CLOSING: |
|---|---|---|---|---|
| Sit in a quiet, comfortable spot with a straight back.<br><br>Set a timer for 15-20 minutes, the typical duration for TM.<br><br>Close your eyes. | Take a few deep breaths to relax your body and clear your mind. | Start repeating your mantra silently. Use 'peace' or 'love' if you don't have a specific one.<br><br>Softly echo the mantra internally. | Let your mind settle into restful alertness naturally.<br><br>If distracted, gently refocus on the mantra. | At the timer's signal, sit quietly for a moment.<br><br>Open your eyes, breathe deeply, then continue with your day. |

The practice of meditation is meant to be effortless and there's no need to try to control your thoughts actively. The mantra serves as a gentle focal point and the process allows your mind to naturally settle into a state of deep rest.

Dr. David H. Rosmarin, assistant professor of psychology at Harvard Medical School and director of the Spirituality and Mental Health Program at McLean Hospital, in Belmont, Mass. says that the research that has been done on prayer shows that prayer may have benefits similar to meditation: It can calm your nervous system, shutting down your fight or flight response. It can make you less reactive to negative emotions and less angry. As the Bible states, "God gives to His beloved in sleep."

To conclude, the study revealed that individuals with high scores in optimism, reflecting a hopeful outlook on the future, experienced significantly lower rates of heart disease, cancer, and mortality compared to those with high scores in pessimism. Remember, every thought holds the potential to shape our path. So, let us embark on our journey with the firm belief that through the cultivation of a positive and mindful mindset, we may not only transform ourselves but also may ripple waves of positive change into the world around us. May the power of belief and mindfulness guide us toward a life rich in purpose, joy, and fulfillment.

# 5.2 ACTIVITY: GENTLE EXERCISE & OPTIMAL 60-MINUTE TRAINING PLAN (5 DAYS/WEEK)

Exercise not only reduces stress levels and boosts cognitive and mental abilities but also builds muscle cells, leading to increased energy. Moreover, it has anti-aging benefits.[33] The anti-inflammatory effects of exercise are one of the key factors in its ability to combat cardiovascular disease, diabetes, certain cancers, neurodegenerative conditions, and more.[34] A study showed that active people had telomeres 140 base pairs longer than inactive ones, appearing years "younger." Larry Tucker of Brigham Young University notes, "Telomeres show cell aging. Active adults are biologically nine years younger than sedentary ones at the same age, a significant difference." [35]

Incorporating moderate physical activity into your routine is essential for overall well-being and supports the detox process. On an average day, people naturally accumulate 3,000 to 6,000 steps through activities like commuting and shopping. To meet the recommended 7,000 to 10,000 daily steps, consider adding 30-40 minutes of walking (3,000 - 4,000 steps). This gentle exercise indirectly aids detoxification, enhances well-being, and provides crucial benefits such as improved oxygen supply for metabolism, better blood flow, enhanced digestion and stress reduction.

However, during detox, it is important not to strain your body with intense exercise routines. Intense workouts can divert energy from the detoxification process, leading to fatigue and weakness. Opt for gentler, more relaxing forms of physical activity, such as Yoga, Pilates, Tai Chi or leisurely walks. Connecting with nature during your walks and taking deep breaths further enhances these benefits by improving oxygen circulation throughout your body.

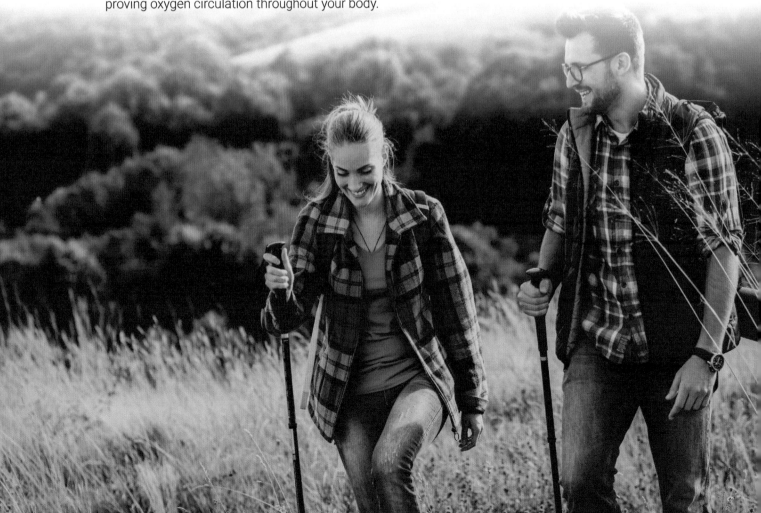

## INCORPORATE MOVEMENT INTO YOUR DAILY LIFE:

✔ Stand or walk while Zooming, calling or reading

✔ Use a height-adjustable computer desk

✔ Opt for stairs over elevators

✔ Park farther away to include more walking

✔ Target 7000-10,000 daily steps

## THE OPTIMUM 60 MINUTE TRAINING PLAN FOR YOUR HEALTH

Target: 5 days per week (90% endurance & 10% strength training / high-intensity interval training (HIIT)

Low-intensity aerobic exercise boosts mitochondrial energy production and burns fat. The ideal workout balances aerobic endurance training and anaerobic muscle building, with 90% being aerobic and only 10% anaerobic.

| DURATION | HEART RATE (beats per minute) |
|----------|-------------------------------|
| 15 min | Resting heart rate + 20 |
| 5 min | Stretching |
| 15 min | Resting heart rate + 25 |
| 5 min | Stretching |
| 15 min | Resting heart rate + 30 |
| 5 min | Stretching |

NOTE: Your resting heart rate is the number of heartbeats per minute when at rest. Check it in the morning after a good night's sleep, before getting out of bed. Keep a record to track improvement.

To summarize, fitness isn't about constant rest or non-stop training. True fitness comes from finding and consistently maintaining the right balance between exercise and rest tailored to your needs.

5.3 LEISURE: ESSENCE OF QUALITY SLEEP AND REST

Ample relaxation, tranquility and a good night's sleep are essential for recovery and rejuvenation. Scientists have extensively explored the advantages of sleep and found that a sufficient duration (7-9 hours) is crucial for immune function, metabolism, memory, learning and reducing mental fatigue. According to the restorative theory, sleep provides the opportunity for the body to repair and replenish cellular components necessary for vital biological functions that may become depleted during waking hours [36, 37]. However, regeneration is only possible without stress. If stress levels are high during sleep, you will not regain energy.

Lack of sleep induces stress, affecting both the mind and body by overstimulating the sympathetic nervous system. Recovering from even a short period of insufficient sleep takes a considerable amount of time, and the lost hours cannot be fully compensated. Sleep deprivation, which affects around 30% of the population sleeping less than 5-6 hours at night, leads to various issues and diseases:

✔ Fatigue, lack of concentration, motivation, creativity and productivity.

✔ Communication problems, emotional disorders, dissatisfaction, unethical behavior and egocentricity.

✔ Cardiovascular diseases, including high blood pressure and tachycardia, due to elevated cortisol levels.

✔ Type 2 diabetes risk increases with insulin resistance, affecting cellular energy.

✔ Overweight issues result from a Leptin/Ghrelin imbalance, leading to increased hunger even after eating.

✔ Lack of sleep raises endocannabinoid levels, triggering cravings.

✔ Increased body-mass-index and adiposity are linked to elevated inflammatory mediators.

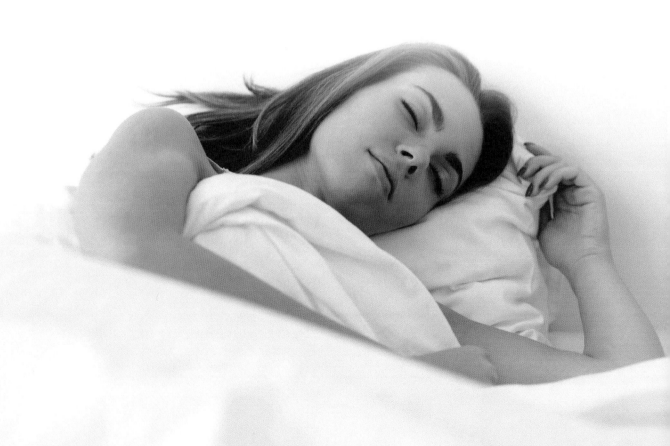

# What might trigger sleep disturbances?

- Night work and LED/blue light from devices delay melatonin release.
- (Ab)use of substances such as caffeine, synthetic stimulants, sleeping pills, and alcohol.
- Travels and jet lag disrupting the preset circadian 24-hour rhythm.
- Consuming too much food late at night, slowing down digestive activity and leading to fermentation or putrefaction gases that intoxicate the liver, causing wakefulness between 1:00 and 3:00 AM.
- Emotional stress from personal problems and fears, coupled with the inability to cope with high personal and societal expectations.
- Information overload, constant communication, and multitasking hinder relaxation and "shutting off".
- Artificial regulation of room temperature.
- Abrupt sleep interruption by alarms.
- Lack of exercise resulting in a lack of oxygen.
- Engaging in physical activity too close to bedtime.

# Guidelines for Quality Sleep[38]

**Bedtime Routine and Environment:**
- Follow a consistent sleep schedule based on circadian rhythm.
- Create a serene sleeping environment with darkness, quiet and cool temperatures (around 65 F / 18 C are ideal).
- Minimize evening blue light exposure from screens.
- Optimize sleep position with a 3-5° angle elevation of the entire bedplane at the head end.
- Choose a gradual wake-up method to prevent shock arousal.

**Pre-Bed Relaxation Techniques:**
- Allow time to unwind with activities like listening to music, reading or mindful meditation.
- Consider strategic napping (20-30 minutes) before 3:00 PM for various benefits.
- Refrain from exercise and drinking liquids 2-3 hours before bedtime.
- Indulging in a warm bath before bedtime can lower your body temperature when you're in bed, promoting a more tranquil and relaxed state, inducing sleepiness.

**Dietary Considerations & Eating Habits:**
- Limit fructose intake, as intolerance may be linked to melatonin deficiency.
- Avoid big meals 3 hours before bedtime to protect REM sleep. Try an 8:16 eating pattern for better HGH (Human Growth Hormone) production, skipping dinner (not breakfast) 2-3 times weekly.
- Avoid caffeine after 2 PM; its effects can last 8 hours.
- Avoid consuming raw food after 4:00 PM, as incomplete digestion at night causes bloating with toxic gases!
- Alcohol before going to bed may help you relax, but too much of it robs you REM sleep.

| WEEKS | 1 | 2 | 3 | 4+ |
|---|---|---|---|---|
| WEIGHT (kg/lbs) | | | | |
| HIPS cm/ inch | | | | |
| WAIST cm/inch (across the belly button) | | | | |
| MORNING SALIVA or URINE PH (7.0-8.0) Target: 7.4-7.5 | | | | |
| RESTING HEART RATE (lower is better) | | | | |
| TONGUE (Scale 1 to 5 from Coated to Pink) | | | | |
| MOOD (Scale 1 to 5 from Sad to Happy) | | | | |
| ENERGY LEVEL (Scale 1 to 5 from Low to High) | | | | |
| SKIN & HAIR (Scale 1 to 5 Improving) | | | | |
| SLEEP (Scale 1 to 5 from Bad to Good) | | | | |
| STRESS LEVEL (Scale 1 to 5 from High to Low) | | | | |
| OTHER (CHOOSE YOUR OWN HEALTH CHALLENGE) | | | | |

NOTE: If you own a blood pressure monitor, remember to also keep a record of your blood pressure readings.

# What are parameters of good health?

## A healthy, flat stomach without intestinal problems and maldigestion.

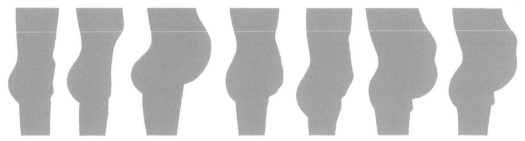

Source: International Society of Mayr Doctors. www.fxmayr.com

**Which abdomen indicates true health?** Exactly, it's the one on the far left.

The second one (from the left) is an empty, hungry abdomen. The third one is excessively bloated with gas and trapped stool. Both the small and large intestines are congested, causing significant pressure on the pelvic organs. In women, this pressure can lead to a forward tilt of the pelvis as a reflex. To protect itself, the body unconsciously adopts a hollow-back posture, often referred to as the duck posture. The fourth person's abdomen is notably flabby and sluggish, while the fifth person's is inflamed. In the sixth and seventh individuals, the abdomen is distended with gas and feces, resulting in variable spinal and postural responses.

In addition, scientific evidence links colon toxicity to skin changes like wrinkles, sagging skin, double chins and pendulous breasts, as well as to conditions like acne, boils, hives, eczema and blemishes, affecting even hair and nails. Detoxifying and improving intestinal health can reverse these signs, unless they've become irreversible. Additionally, toxin damage manifests itself in external signs progressing from the puffy stage to the flaccid stage and ultimately to skin thinning, indicating different phases of toxicity.

## In conclusion, achieving good health involves:

✔ Consuming a diverse range of foods.
✔ Maintaining an upright posture with relaxed muscles.
✔ Ensuring detoxification of cells and the matrix.
✔ Optimizing oxygen supply to cells.
✔ Minimizing inflammatory activity while enhancing immune system resilience.
✔ Reducing insulin resistance to the lowest possible level (a key factor in type II Diabetes).
✔ Aiming for optimal vitality and athletic performance.
✔ Cultivating more happiness and balance.

In summary, the human body is inherently acid-producing. This acid production can lead to a condition called metabolic acidosis. To balance this, it is important to follow a diet that increases alkalinity.

# 5.5.1 12 GOLDEN RULES FOR UPGRADED HEALTH

**1**

**DIVERSITY is everything!**

Eat a variety of foods as a diverse microbiome is directly linked to good health and longevity. It will also help you avoid intolerances as intolerances occur when we eat too much of the same food too often. The only exception to this routine is during the initial 2-week phase of our 3-week program, where we purposefully give a rest to the digestive system by allowing a period of monotony.

**2**

**A BALANCED MEAL OF 70% ALKALINE & 30% ACIDIC INGREDIENTS**

Maintaining a balance between acids and bases is vital for metabolism. Strive for a diet that is 70% alkaline and 30% acidic (see table below). Alkaline-rich foods help counteract excess acid from poor eating, stress, and inactivity. Prioritize vegetables in your lunch and dinner, aiming for three times more vegetables than fruit! EAT RAW FOODS ONLY BEFORE 16:00 - never in the evening! Risk of fermentation thus bloating with toxic gases! Avoid "Mineral - stealers": white flour products, sugar, too much coffee, alcohol, chocolate, sweet snacks.

**3**

**ONLY ORGANIC, ALL NATURAL**

Only consume clean, organic / natural, locally grown, nutrient dense ingredients (ideally in season). Sun-ripened ingredients are key as their bio-photons have a positive influence on cell renewal, regeneration and fat reduction. AVOID: preservatives, soup cubes, artificial sweeteners such as aspartame, flavor enhancers, additives and artificial coloring, maltodextrin, citric acid and carrageenan.

**4**

**INCREASE FERMENTED VEGETABLES**

Fermented foods provide many health benefits such as antioxidant, anti-microbial, anti-fungal, anti-inflammatory, anti-diabetic activity. Eat fermented vegetables (i.e. sauerkraut, kimchi, kefir etc. ) increasing step by step targeting 100 – 500g / day before 16:00 => effective against food cravings as they are feeding beneficial bacteria (actinobacteria) in the gut.

**5**

**INCREASE FIBER**

Enjoy eating the right fiber (barley, chickpeas, edamame, lentils, quinoa, peas, berries, pears, artichokes, avocados, nuts, carrots, sweet potatoes etc.). Reduce the amount of coarse grains as finely ground grains can help you avoid feeling bloated.

## 6 EAT SLOWLY FOR EATING LESS

Chew your food at least 20-40 times until the food is liquified to promote its digestion! When you eat slowly, you will not overeat, thanks to leptin release after 15 minutes and you will be able to adjust to the natural feeling of satiety (stop eating when the feeling of fullness occurs). GOLDEN RULE! Eat breakfast like an emperor, lunch like a king and dinner like a beggar (preferably only a soup or skip dinner during intermittent fasting days)! Allow 5 hours between meals. Eating at the right time facilitates optimal metabolism. TIP! To curb cravings and hunger, spoon evening liquids i.e. vegetable broth, even tea, instead of drinking them. This helps you feel fuller and can help cut calories!

## 7 DRINK MORE WATER

The first sip of water that you drink in the morning activates your entire digestive system and kidneys. Consume 2-3 liters of quality spring water (non-carbonated), caffeine-free herbal teas and vegetable broth daily, spreading intake throughout the day, but avoiding liquids 30 minutes before and after meals, as not to dilute the gastric juices for optimal digestion. Aim for 2/3 of the daily intake in the morning and 1/3 in the afternoon. Avoid fruit juices.

## 8 WEEKLY INTERMITTENT FASTING

Practice intermittent fasting (16 hours of fasting – skipping dinner): Skip dinner 3 days a week during the 21-day detox and continue 2 + evenings each week thereafter for anti-aging benefits as the growth hormone (somatotropin) and autophagy get activated when we are fasting for min. 16 hours overnight. Growth hormone helps to break down fat and build muscle, lengthens the life of cells and promotes DNA repair mechanisms in the body.

## 9 DAILY MOVING / EXERCISE

Walk 7,000 - 10,000 steps daily to support digestion and prevent constipation. Optimal health involves a 40 - 60 minute exercise plan, 5 days a week, with 90% aerobic and 10% anaerobic exercises for improved endurance and muscle building. Refer to Section 5.2 Activity for guidance. Additionally, keep in mind the importance of taking deep breaths, as they play a crucial role in various metabolic processes, including detoxification.

## 10 LESS SUGAR

SUGAR - max 1g/day. Choose natural sweeteners (honey, coconut palm sugar, currants and raisins, maple syrup) over artificial ones like aspartame and saccharin, which should be avoided. Be mindful even with healthy fruit sugars from fruit or juice concentrate (like apple, pear or agave) and use them sparingly.

## 11 DAILY SUPPLEMENTS

Because of nutrient-depleted soils, it is advisable to incorporate supplements into our diet, with a preference for plant-based options to enhance absorption. Alongside a comprehensive multivitamin and multimineral supplement, consider adding extra Vitamin D, prebiotics, probiotics, digestive bitters to stimulate enzymes, Omega-3 fatty acids (2000 mg EPA/DHA), and 2 teaspoons of linseed/flaxseed oil (abundant in ALA). Discover highly concentrated plant-based supplements at UPGRADERS.com. Toxins block nutrient absorption, affecting your overall health, beauty, vitality and well-being. Thus, regular detoxification (1 to 3 times a year) is highly recommended.

## 12 CUT BACK ON ALCOHOL

Cutting alcohol is crucial for weight management and health in general, as already one glass halts fat burning for 24 hours. Two nightly beer bottles can add up to an extra 44 pounds (22 kg) annually, while two glasses of wine daily may contribute 22 pounds (10 kg). Limit alcohol to 2-3 times a week, with one serving of red wine (0.2L or 6.7 Oz) or beer (0.5L or 16.9 Oz).

# 5.5.2. UPGRADERS® METHOD FOOD PYRAMID

## NUTRITION = HEALTHY DIETARY CHOICES x EFFICIENT DIGESTION

---

### HEALTHY DIETARY CHOICES =
### A BALANCED MEAL OF 70% ALKALINE & 30% ACIDIC INGREDIENTS

Opt for clean, organic, locally-sourced, nutrient-rich and sun-ripened ingredients, ideally in season, as bio-photons in food enhance cell renewal, regeneration and fat reduction.

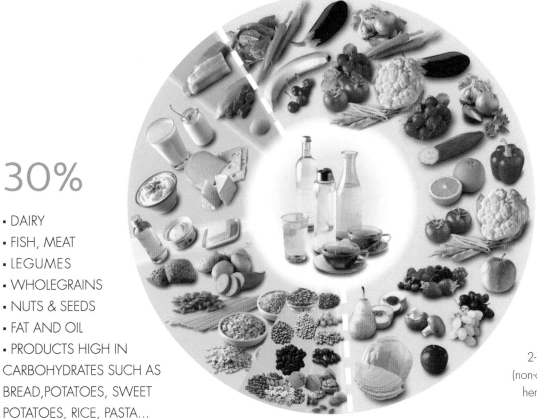

**70%**

2/3 VEGETABLES
1/3 FRUIT

**30%**

- DAIRY
- FISH, MEAT
- LEGUMES
- WHOLEGRAINS
- NUTS & SEEDS
- FAT AND OIL
- PRODUCTS HIGH IN CARBOHYDRATES SUCH AS BREAD,POTATOES, SWEET POTATOES, RICE, PASTA...

**LIQUIDS**

2-3 liters of spring water (non-carbonated), caffeine-free herbal teas and vegetable broth daily.

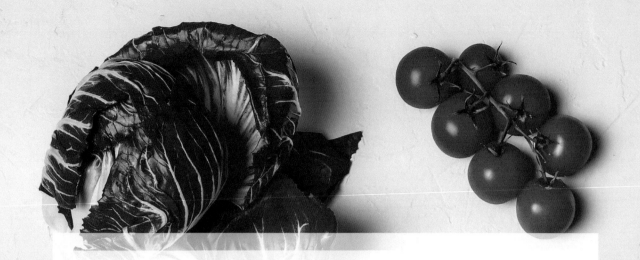

## EFFICIENT DIGESTION =

Use Hand Dimensions for Portions: Use hand sizes to measure food for balanced meals without counting calories.

———————————————

Chew Well to Aid Digestion: Chew each bite 20-40 times for better digestion and to naturally control appetite. Stop eating when the feeling of fullness occurs!

———————————————

Meal Size & Timing: To boost metabolism, opt for a hearty breakfast, a moderate lunch, and a light dinner, spaced 5 hours apart.

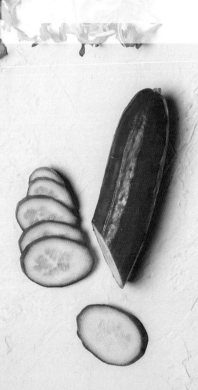

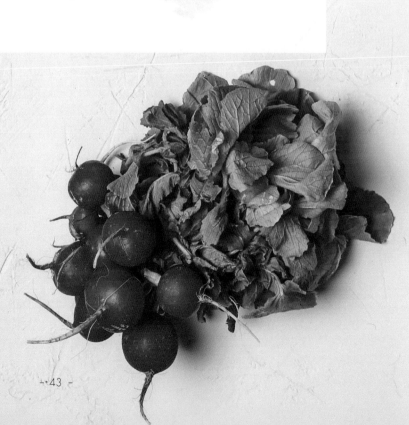

# 5.5.3 ALKALINE & ACIDIC INGREDIENTS: YOUR SHOPPING COMPANION

**The primary rule is to create balanced meals with 70% alkaline and 30% acidic ingredients.**

Maintaining a balance between acids and bases is vital for metabolism. Strive for a diet that is 70% alkaline and 30% acidic (see table below). Alkaline-rich foods help counteract excess acid from poor eating, stress and inactivity. Achieving a healthy acid-base balance, indicated by a saliva pH range of 7.0-8.0, plays a pivotal role in fortifying the body's immune system. This balance serves as a cornerstone for overall well-being, empowering the body to resist various health challenges and supporting your path to vibrant health.

## The At-A-Glance Acid/Alkaline Food List

EAT MORE ← ————————————————————————— → EAT LESS

CAN BE INCLUDED IN YOUR 20% ACID

| Highly Alkaline | Moderately Alkaline | Mildly Alkaline | Neutral/ Mildly Acidic | Moderately Acidic | Highly Acidic |
|---|---|---|---|---|---|
| Broccoli | Avocado | Almond Milk | Amaranth | Apple | Alcohol |
| Cucumber | Beetroot | Avocado Oil | Black Beans | Apricot | Artificial Sweeteners |
| Grasses | Beans | Artichokes | Brazil Nuts | Banana | Beef |
| Green Drinks | Butter Beans | Asparagus | Cantaloupe | Blackberry | Black Tea |
| Himalayan Salt | Capsicum/Pepper | Brussels Sprouts | Currants | Blueberry | Cheese |
| Kale | Cabbage | Buckwheat | Chickpeas/ | Brown Rice | Chicken |
| Kelp | Celery | Cauliflower | Garbanzos | Butter | Coffee |
| Parsley | Collard/Spring | Carrot | Freshwater Wild | Cranberry | Cocoa |
| pH 9.5 Alkaline Water | Chia/Salba | Chives | Fish | Fresh Juice | Dairy |
| Spinach | Endive | Courgette/Zucchini | Fresh Dates | Grapes | Dried Fruit |
| Sprouted Beans | Greens | Coconut Oil | Grapeseed Oil | Ketchup | Eggs |
| Sprouts (Soy, Alfalfa) | Garlic | Coconut | Hazel Nuts | Mayonnaise | Farmed Fish |
| Sea Vegetables | Ginger | Flax Oil/ Udo's Oil | Hemp | Mango | Fruit Juice (Sweetened) |
| (Kelp) | Green Beans | Grapefruit | Kidney Beans | Mangosteen | Honey |
| | Lettuce | Goat Milk | Millet | Oats | Jam |
| | Mustard Greens | Herbs & Spices | Nectarine | Ocean Fish | Jelly |
| | Okra | Leeks | Oats/Oatmeal | Orange | Mustard |
| | Onion | Lentils | Pecan Nuts | Peach | Miso |
| | Radish | Mushroooms | Plum | Papaya | Pork |
| | Red Onion | New Baby Potatoes | Protein | Pineapple | Rice Syrup |
| | Rocket/Arugula | Other Beans & | Rice/Rice Milk | Strawberry | Soy Sauce |
| | Quinoa | Legumes | Soy/Soy Milk | Rye Bread | Shellfish |
| | Soy Beans | Peas | Soybeans | Wheat | Syrup |
| | Tomato | Rhubarb | Spelt | Wholemeal Bread | Vinegar |
| | Lemon | Swede | Seitan | Wild Rice | Yeast |
| | Lime | Tofu | Sunflower Oil | Wholemeal Pasta | |
| | White Haricot | Watercress | Sweet Cherry | | |
| | | | Watermelon | | |

# The Detailed List of Alkaline Foods

Eat these alkaline foods freely! Try to incorporate as many as you can into your daily diet...

## Vegetables

| | |
|---|---|
| Asparagus | Garlic |
| Basil | Green Beans |
| Beetroot | Kale |
| Brussels Sprouts | Kelp |
| Broccoli | Lettuce |
| Broad Beans | Mushrooms |
| Chard | New Potato |
| Cabbage | Onion |
| Celery | Parsley |
| Cucumber | Peas |
| Coriander | Pumpkin |
| Cauliflower | Radish |
| Carrot | Runner Beans |
| Chilli | Snowpeas |
| Capsicum/Pepper | String Beans |
| Courgette/Zucchini | Spinach |
| Collards | Sweet Potato |
| Chives | Wakame |
| Dandelion | Watercress |
| Eggplant/ | |
| Aubergine | |
| Endive | |

## Fruit

Avocado
Fresh Coconut
Grapefruit
Lemon
Lime
Tomato

## Grains & Beans

| | |
|---|---|
| Amaranth | Mung Beans |
| Buckwheat | Navy Beans |
| Brown Rice | Pinto Beans |
| Chia/Salba | Quinoa |
| Kamut | Red Beans |
| Lentils | Spelt |
| Lima Beans | Soy Beans |
| Millet | White Beans |

## Grasses

Barley Grass
Dog Grass
Kamut Grass
Oat Grass
Shave Grass
Wheatgrass

## Nuts & Seeds

Almonds
Coconut
Flax Seeds
Pumpkin Seeds
Sesame Seeds
Sunflower Seeds

## Oils

Avocado Oil
Coconut Oil
Flax Oil
Olive Oil
Udo's Oil

## Breads

Sprouted Bread
Sprouted Wraps
Gluten/Yeast Free
Breads & Wraps

## Other

Almond Milk
Alkaline Water
Goat Milk
Herbal Tea
Tofu

## Sprouts

| | | |
|---|---|---|
| Alfalfa Sprouts | Kamut Sprouts | Spelt Sprouts |
| Amaranth Sprouts | Mung Bean Sprouts | Soy Sprouts |
| Broccoli Sprouts | Quinoa Sprouts | |
| Fenugreek Sprouts | Radish Sprouts | |

# The Detailed List of Acid Foods

Try to avoid these foods and drinks, and try to keep to a maximum of 20% of your diet

## Meat

| | |
|---|---|
| Bacon | Pork |
| Beef | Rabbit |
| Clams | Sausage |
| Corned Beef | Scallops |
| Eggs | Shellfish |
| Fish | Shrimp |
| Lamb | Tuna |
| Lobster | Turkey |
| Mussels | Venison |
| Organ Meats | Veal |
| Oyster | |

## Fruit

| | |
|---|---|
| Apple | Orange |
| Apricot | Pineapple |
| Berries | Plum |
| Cantaloupe | Peach |
| Cranberries | Pear |
| Currants | Prunes |
| Dates | Raisins |
| Grapes | Raspberries |
| Honeydew | Strawberries |
| Mango | Tropical Fruits |
| Melon | |

## Drinks

| | |
|---|---|
| Alcohol | Flavoured |
| Black Tea | Water |
| Cocoa | Green Tea |
| Coffee | Milk |
| Colas | Pasteurized |
| Carbonated | Juice |
| Water | Sports Drinks |
| Decaffeinated | Tap Water |
| Drinks | |
| Energy Drinks | |

## Nuts & Seeds

Brazil Nuts
Chestnuts
Cashews
Hazelnuts
Macadamia Nuts
Peanuts
Pecans
Pistachios
Walnuts

## Sweeteners

| | |
|---|---|
| Artificial | Processed |
| Sweeteners | Sugar |
| Carob | Saccharine |
| Corn Syrup | Sucrose |
| Fructose | Sucralose |
| Honey | |
| Maple Syrup | |

## Dairy & Eggs

| | |
|---|---|
| Butter | Sour |
| Cheese | Cream |
| Cottage | Whey |
| Cheese | Yogurt |
| Eggs | |
| Ice Cream | |
| Milk | |

## Other

| | |
|---|---|
| Biscuits | Noodles |
| Candy | Pastas |
| Cigarettes | Pizza |
| Chocolate | Rice |
| Chips | White Breads |
| Drugs | |
| Miso | |

## Sauce

Ketchup
Mayonnaise
Mustard
Pickles
Soy Sauce
Tabasco
Tamari
Vinegar
Wasabi

## Oils!

Cooked Oil
Margarine

# 5.5.4 DAILY DETOX SCHEDULE FOR 21 DAYS

Our plan rejuvenates your cells, rebalances pH, and maximizes
nutrient absorption for upgraded health.

| TIME | TASK | GUIDELINES |
|---|---|---|
| WAKE UP | Measure first morning urine and saliva pH (before meal & before brushing your teeth) with pH PAPER STRIPS | Measure at the beginning and at the end of the program. Follow the **UPGRADERS® 21-day Health & Beauty Pro Detox & Intermittent Fasting Set** guidelines. |
| | Take the CLEANSE supplement as directed. | The right concentration of the cleanse supplement effectively purifies the gut and liver. Follow the **UPGRADERS® 21-day Health & Beauty Pro Detox & Intermittent Fasting Set** supplement guidelines.<br><br>RECOMMENDED! Kickstart your digestive system with a quick stretch or outdoor walk / exercise (~ 20 minutes) after taking Magnesium Citrate and before breakfast. |
| BREAKFAST 7:00 - 9:00 | Check Food Guidelines and BREAKFAST recipes. Follow UPGRADERS® supplement directions. | IMPORTANT! Keep 5-hour gaps between meals. |
| 10:00-11:00 | Adhere to UPGRADERS® supplement instructions. | A balanced acid-base ratio is crucial for optimal metabolism and autophagy, the cell recycling and renewal process central to anti-aging. |

| TIME | TASK | GUIDELINES |
|---|---|---|
| **LUNCH**<br>**12:00 - 14:00** | Check Food Guidelines and LUNCH recipes. Follow UPGRADERS® supplement directions. | RECOMMENDED! After lunch: energize your metabolism with a 5-minute rest and a quick ~ 20 minute walk/exercise. |
| **DINNER**<br>**17:00 - 19:00** | Check Food Guidelines and DINNER recipes. Follow UPGRADERS® supplement directions.<br><br>INTERMITTENT FASTING: Begin by skipping dinner for the first 3 evenings of the program, and then continue with 3 evenings a week during the 21 days. Afterward, aim for 2 or more evenings a week. | INTERMITTENT FASTING (no food for min. 16 hours) is a great anti-aging method as the human growth hormone (HCG) and autophagy get activated when we are fasting for min. 16 hours overnight. If you want to skip a meal, it is better to skip dinner instead of breakfast. This way, your stomach will be empty overnight, allowing HCG production and repair work.<br><br>TIP! To curb cravings and hunger, spoon evening liquids i.e. vegetable broth, even tea, instead of drinking them. This helps you feel fuller and can help cut calories! |
| **20:00 - 21:00** | Adhere to UPGRADERS® supplement instructions. | Support nightly liver regeneration. |
| **BEDTIME**<br>**~22:00** | At the latest at 22:00 go to sleep | Regular early bedtime and sleep before midnight are crucial for deep sleep. Avoid burdening the autonomic nervous system and thus negatively impacting the regeneration process: TV, mobile phone, bright and blue light, hot baths.<br><br>RECOMMENDED! Meditation provides calm, peace, and balance for emotional and physical health. Explore Transcendental Meditation on YouTube, a science-backed method. |

# 5.5.5 21-DAY DETOX FOOD GUIDELINES AND BEYOND

This program focuses on savoring your favorite dishes crafted from high-quality, organic, seasonal ingredients cooked gently to retain nutrients.

## DETOX WEEKS 1-2
### Cleanse & Simplify

| NO GO | ENJOY |
|---|---|
| NO COW MILK DAIRY | Gluten-free sheep and goat milk and "milk" from oat, almond, coconut, rice, soy and chestnut / soft cheese / yogurt. Pasture-raised eggs. Butter and ghee are acceptable. |
| NO GLUTEN | Gluten free oats, millet, buckwheat, quinoa, rice, corn, amaranth |
| NO RAW FOODS – salads, fruits, raw juices or smoothies | Herbs and sprouts as meal toppings. Lime, lemon, olives. |
| NO FERMENTED VEGETABLES | All cooked vegetables, vegetable spreads, hummus, vegetable broth |
| NO CAFFEINE | 1 unsweetened espresso / day (if headache or low blood pressure), herbal teas |
| NO ALCOHOL | |
| NO NICOTINE | |
| NO SUGAR, ARTIFICIAL SWEETENERS | Almond butter, a little honey or 80% dark chocolate (in the morning or directly after lunch) |
| NO NUTS | Use chia, flax, sunflower, pumpkin seeds |
| NO MEAT | |
| NO FISH | |
| NO PROCESSED FOODS | Organic / all natural / seasonal |

# POST-DETOX WEEK 3 & BEYOND
## Sustain & Diversify

| LIMIT | ENJOY |
|---|---|
| LIMIT COW MILK DAIRY | Gluten-free sheep and goat milk and "milk" from oat,almond,coconut,rice, soy and chestnut / soft cheese / yogurt. Free - range eggs. FERMENTED DAIRY: kefir, yogurt. HIGH FAT COW MILK: Quark, heavy whipping cream, butter, ghee. |
| LOW GLUTEN | Gluten free oats, millet, buckwheat, quinoa, rice, corn,amaranth. LOW GLUTEN: Rye, Durum wheat, Spelt |
| NO RAW FOODS AFTER 16:00 | Slowly introduce seasonal raw foods (salad, berries, fruit) |
| | 70% VEGETABLES +FERMENTED VEGETABLES<br>All cooked vegetables, vegetable spreads, hummus, vegetable / bone broth. Slowly introduce Sauerkraut juice, kimchi. |
| LIMIT CAFFEINE | Max. 2 espressos / day, green tea |
| LIMIT ALCOHOL | Max. 2-3 x week with one serving of red wine (0.2L or 6.7Oz) or beer (0.5L or 16.9 Oz) |
| NO NICOTINE | Cut back or as little as absolutely necessary |
| LIMIT SUGAR | Almond butter, a little honey or 80% dark chocolate (in the morning or directly after lunch). Max. 1g/day |
| FEW NUTS per day | Use chia, flax, sunflower, pumpkin seeds. Slowly introduce nuts (start with almonds). |
| LEAN MEAT (1-2 x week) | Fresh turkey, chicken, veal, lamb, beef or cured slices of beef / veal or smoked venison |
| FISH (1- 3 x week) | Fresh filet of trout, pike, perch, plaice, char, sole, salmon or smoked trout or salmon filet |
| NO PROCESSED FOODS | Organic / all natural / seasonal |

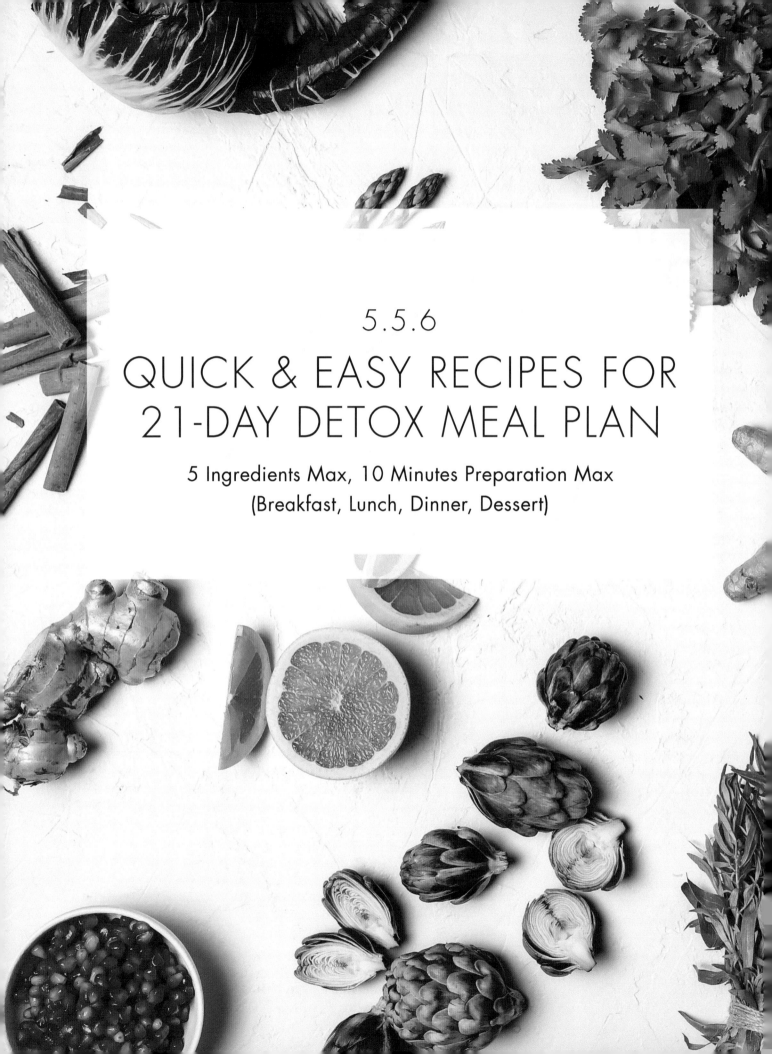

# 5.5.6

# QUICK & EASY RECIPES FOR 21-DAY DETOX MEAL PLAN

## 5 Ingredients Max, 10 Minutes Preparation Max
## (Breakfast, Lunch, Dinner, Dessert)

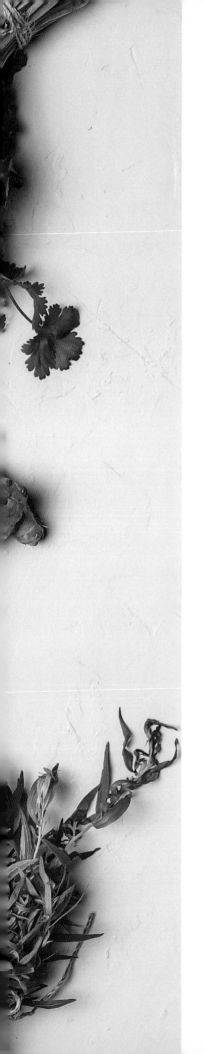

# BREAKFAST

# LUNCH

# DINNER

# DESSERT

# 21-DAY DETOX MEAL PLAN

## DETOX WEEKS 1-2
## Cleanse & Simplify

Select one option for breakfast, lunch, and dinner from the provided sample recipes. Please note that these are just examples, and you're welcome to customize your meals according to the 70% alkaline and 30% acidic ingredients principle.

| BREAKFAST 7:00 - 9:00 | LUNCH 12:00-14:00 (5 hours after breakfast) | DINNER 17:00-19:00 (5 hours after lunch) |
|---|---|---|

### BREAKFAST 7:00 - 9:00

1.1 AVOCADO SPREAD ON GLUTEN FREE TOAST

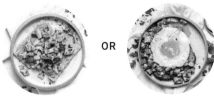

OR

1.2. VEGETABLE SPREAD ON GLUTEN-FREE TOAST

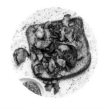

1.3. SOFT CHEESE SPREAD ON GLUTEN-FREE TOAST

2.1. GLUTEN FREE OATMEAL WITH ALMOND BUTTER

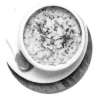

2.2. GLUTEN FREE OVERNIGHT OATS

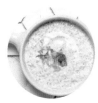

3. BLISS PARFAIT

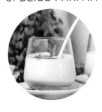

### LUNCH 12:00-14:00 (5 hours after breakfast)

4.1. SEASONAL VEGETABLE MEDLEY WITH FETA

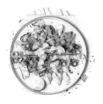

4.2. REFRESHING SEASONAL VEGETABLES AND POTATO MEDLEY

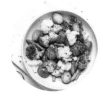

4.4. TOFU WITH RIBBON VEGETABLES

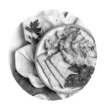

4.7 BEAN MEDLEY WITH SMOKED TOFU

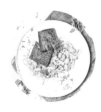

5.1. BROWN RICE PASTA

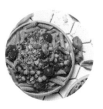

### DINNER 17:00-19:00 (5 hours after lunch)

6.1 ENERGIZING PEA SOUP

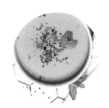

6.2 CALMING PUMPKIN SOUP

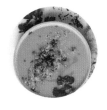

6.3 CARROT GINGER SOUP

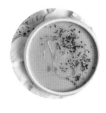

6.4 VITALITY BEETROOT SOUP

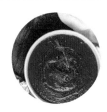

# POST-DETOX WEEK 3 & BEYOND
## Sustain & Diversify

## MEALS FROM WEEKS 1-2 ✚ THE OPTIONS BELOW

| BREAKFAST 7:00 - 9:00 | LUNCH 12:00-14:00 (5 hours after breakfast) | DINNER 17:00-19:00 (5 hours after lunch) |
|---|---|---|

### BREAKFAST 7:00 - 9:00

1.1 AVOCADO SPREAD ON GLUTEN FREE TOAST

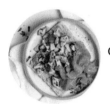 OR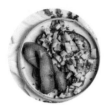

2.1. GLUTEN FREE OATMEAL WITH ALMOND BUT TER

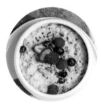

2.2. GLUTEN FREE OVERNIGHT OATS

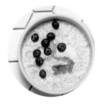

3. BLISS PARFAIT

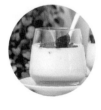

### LUNCH 12:00-14:00 (5 hours after breakfast)

4.3. TANTALIZING A SPARAGUS WITH MEATBALLS

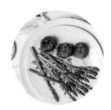

4.5. WILD SALMON WITH RIBBON VEGETABLES

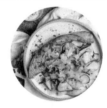

4.6 SAVORY PANCAKES WITH ARTICHOKE HEARTS

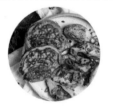

### DINNER 17:00-19:00 (5 hours after lunch)

6.5 IMMUNE-BOOSTING MUSHROOM BOUILLON with FLATBREAD

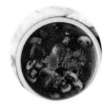

7.1 CHICKEN WITH SPROUTS AND GREENS

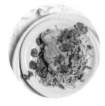

7.2. SOOTHING STEAMED FISH & VEGETABLES

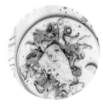

7.3. CHILEAN SEA BASS WITH BABY VEGGIE STIR-FRY

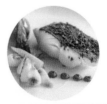

## DESSERT (only after lunch!)

8. FRUIT FRENZY COMPOTE

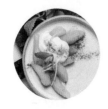

9. DARK CHOCOLATE RASPBERRY DELIGHT

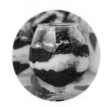

10. DARK CHOCOLATE MOUSSE

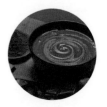

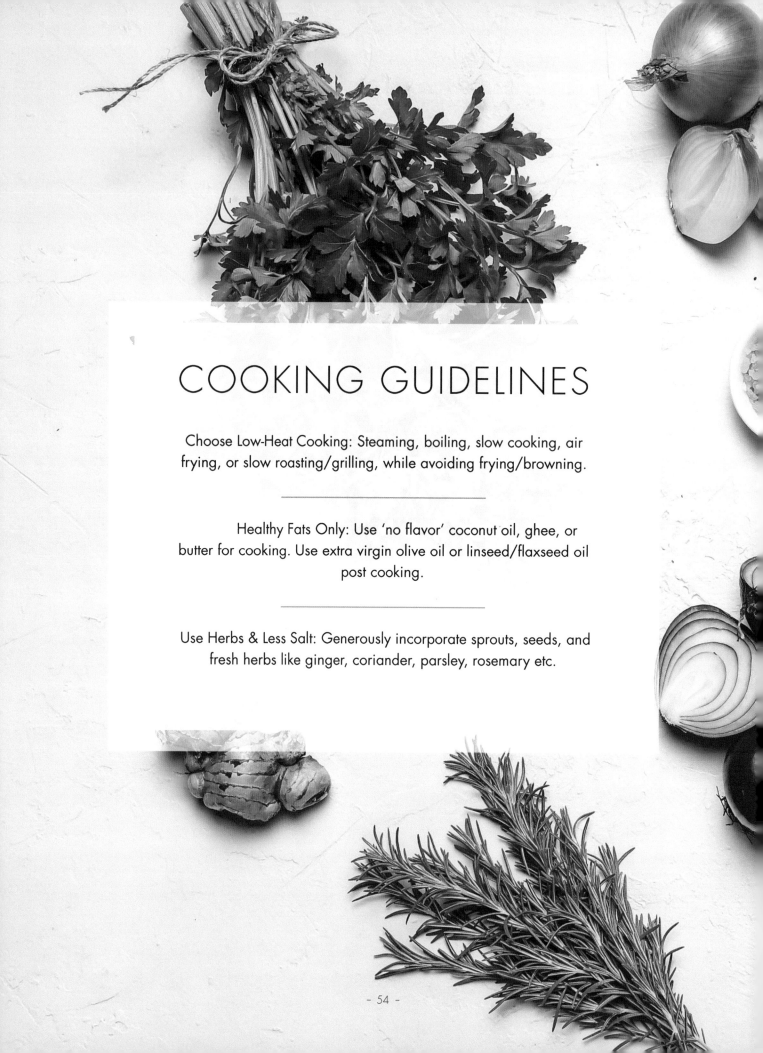

# COOKING GUIDELINES

Choose Low-Heat Cooking: Steaming, boiling, slow cooking, air frying, or slow roasting/grilling, while avoiding frying/browning.

---

Healthy Fats Only: Use 'no flavor' coconut oil, ghee, or butter for cooking. Use extra virgin olive oil or linseed/flaxseed oil post cooking.

---

Use Herbs & Less Salt: Generously incorporate sprouts, seeds, and fresh herbs like ginger, coriander, parsley, rosemary etc.

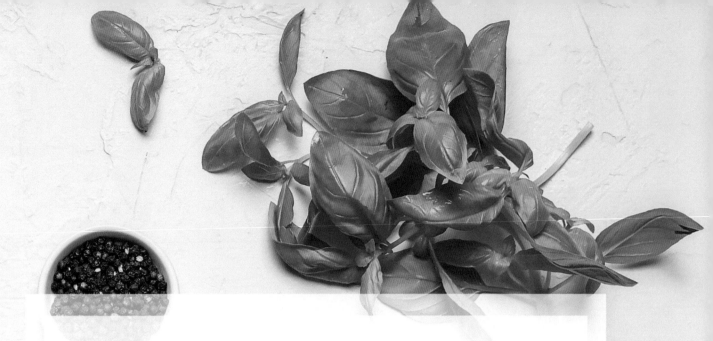

# A CLASSIC SET OF BASICS

A 'classic set of basics' that you should always have at home
(not counted in the 5-ingredient list):

- ✔ ghee (clarified butter), butter, or flavorless refined coconut oil for cooking
- ✔ spices: Himalayan sea salt, black pepper
- ✔ optional spices: curry, ground cumin, and/or red chili flakes
- ✔ extra virgin olive oil (only used cold)
- ✔ linseed / flaxseed oil (anti-inflammatory)
- ✔ balsamic vinegar
- ✔ the 'allium' family: garlic, yellow onion
- ✔ herbs: cilantro, parsley, basil, mint
- ✔ lime and/or lemon
- ✔ honey

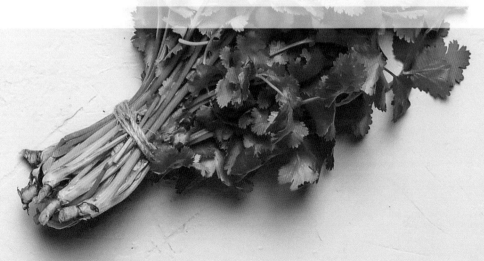

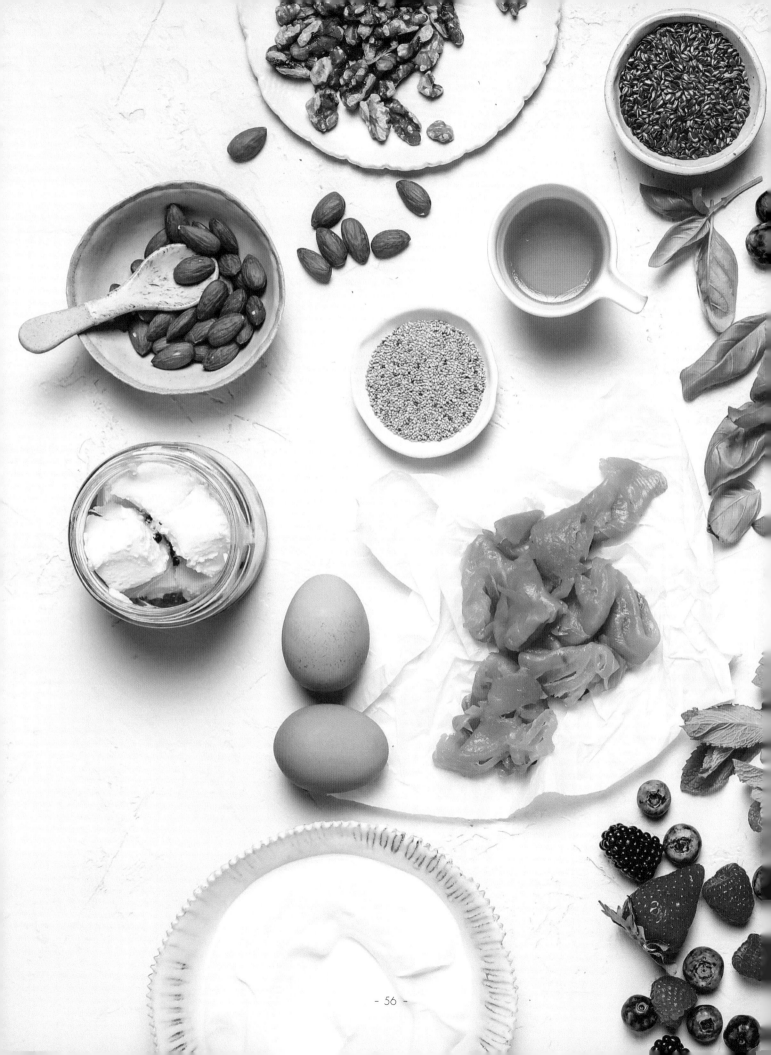

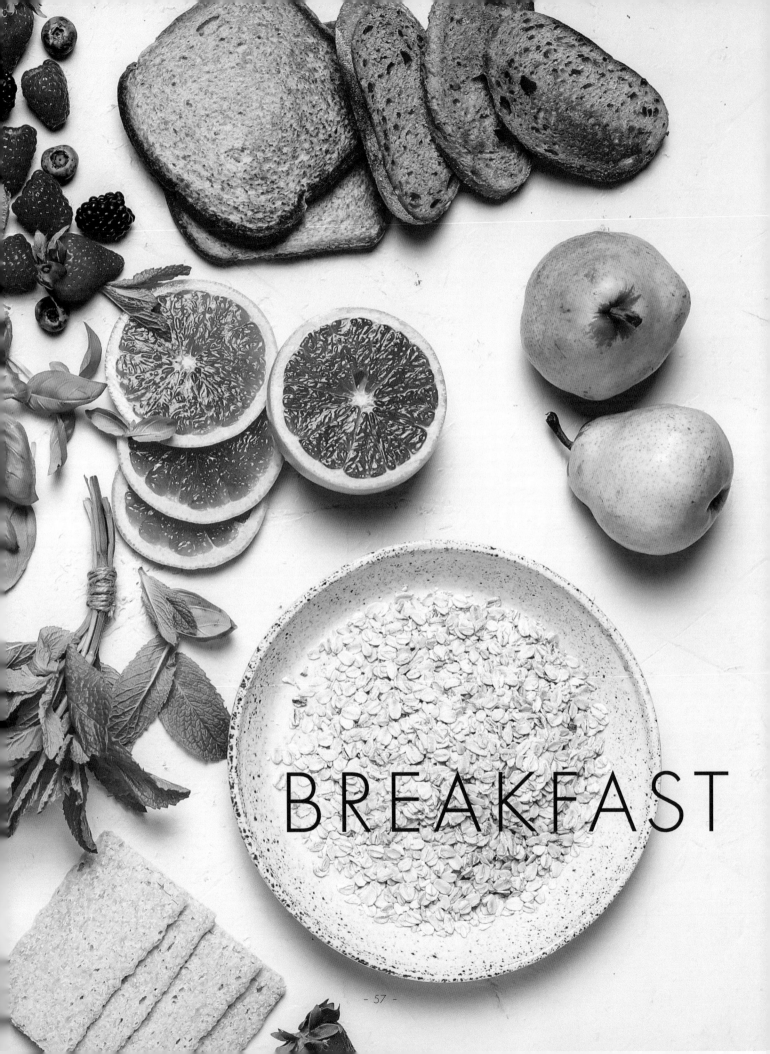

BREAKFAST

# 1. GLUTEN FREE TOAST (or CRISPBREAD) WITH SPREADS

## 1.1 AVOCADO SPREAD ON GLUTEN-FREE TOAST

**4 servings**

- gluten free buckwheat bread (or crispbread)
- 2 ripe avocados
- salt, red chili flakes
- lime juice
- chopped cilantro
- 1 teaspoon of linseed / flaxseed or extra virgin olive oil
- optional: sprouts for garnish

STEP 1: Toast a slice of gluten-free buckwheat bread in a toaster. Alternative: Use gluten free crispbread (chickpea, lentil, quinoa)

STEP 2: Prepare the spread by peeling and pitting the avocados, then cut into pieces or mash the pulp with a fork. Season it to your liking with salt, freshly squeezed lime juice, and chopped cilantro. Sprinkle red chili flakes and garnish with cilantro leaves (optional: add sprouts). For an additional Omega-3 boost, drizzle a dash of linseed/flaxseed or olive oil.

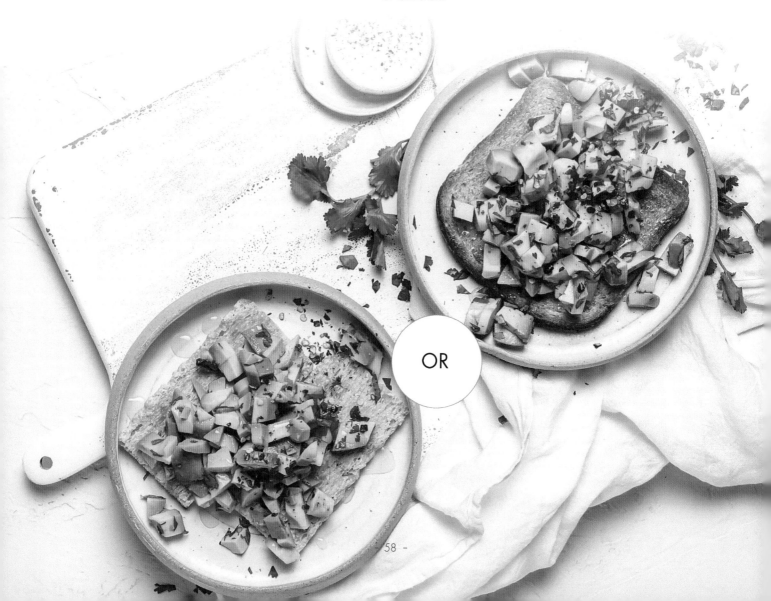

OR

## VARIATIONS TO TRY:

### EGGS

Boil an egg for 5-6 minutes until soft-boiled, season with salt and pepper, and serve it as a delightful side dish. Alternatively, fry an egg sunny-side up and place it on top of the toast for a satisfying variation.

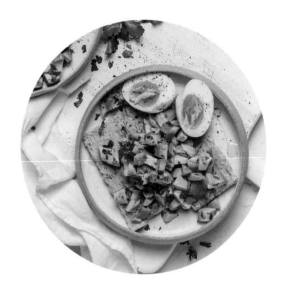

### SALMON

Top your avocado toast with a slice of smoked salmon (or smoked trout) filet.

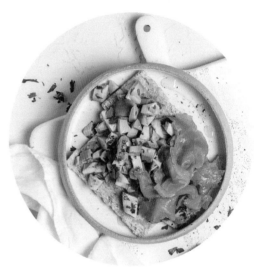

### BEEF, VEAL OR SMOKED VENISON

Enhance your avocado toast with a cured slice of beef, veal or smoked venison.

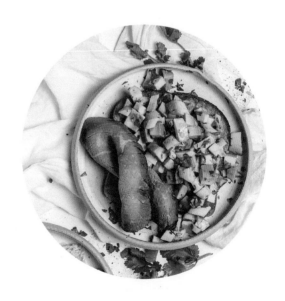

## 1.2. VEGETABLE SPREAD ON GLUTEN-FREE TOAST

**4 servings**

- *gluten free buckwheat bread (or crispbread)*
- *salt, pepper*
- *previous night's cooked veggies (zucchini, eggplant)*
- *chopped sun-dried tomatoes*
- *pesto*
- *chopped cilantro*
- *1 teaspoon of extra virgin olive oil*

STEP 1: Toast a slice of gluten-free buckwheat bread in a toaster. Alternative: Use gluten free crispbread (chickpea, lentil, quinoa)

STEP 2: Dice leftover cooked vegetables (zucchini, eggplant) or puree it in a blender from the night before, season with pesto, salt, pepper, sun-dried tomatoes, and cilantro. Add a drizzle of olive oil for a mediterranean-inspired spread.

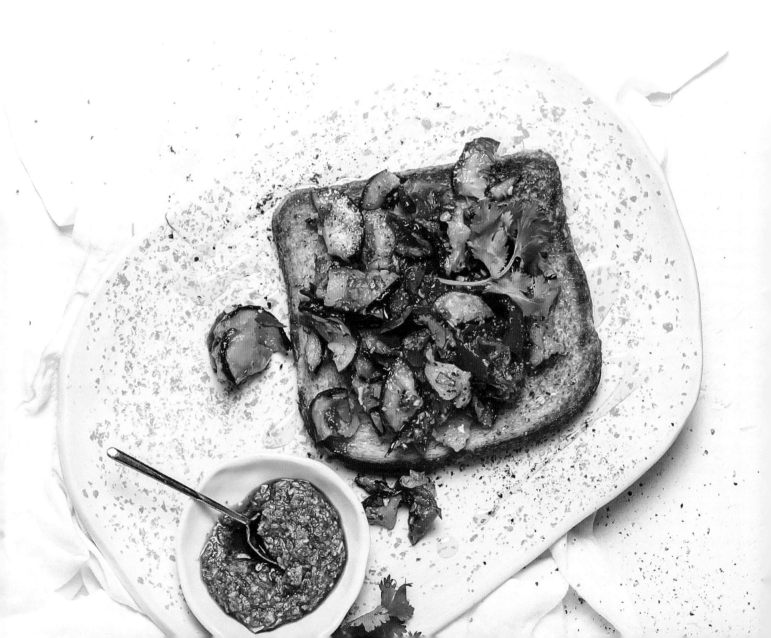

# 1.3. SOFT CHEESE SPREAD ON GLUTEN-FREE TOAST

**4 servings**

- *gluten free buckwheat bread (or crispbread)*
- *salt, pepper*
- *250g (9 oz) soft sheep or goat cheese*
- *few chopped olives*
- *chopped cilantro or parsley*
- *1 teaspoon of linseed / flaxseed or extra virgin olive oil*

STEP 1: Toast a slice of gluten-free buckwheat bread in a toaster. Alternative: Use gluten free crispbread (chickpea, lentil, quinoa)

STEP 2: Prepare the spread by mashing the soft sheep (or goat) cheese with a fork. Season it to your liking with salt, pepper, chopped olives, and cilantro (or parsley). Top it with additional olive pieces and garnish with cilantro leaves. For an extra Omega-3 boost, drizzle a dash of linseed/flaxseed or olive oil.

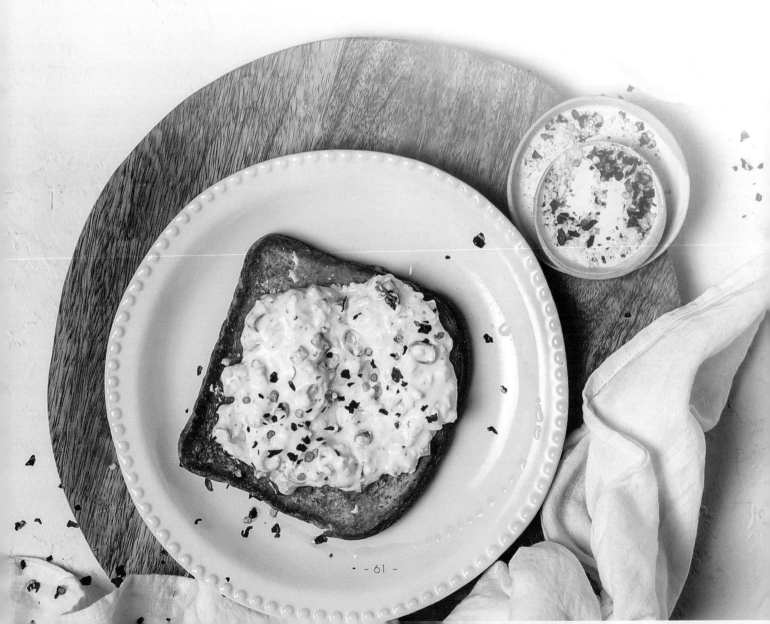

# 2. GLUTEN FREE OATS

## 2.1. GLUTEN FREE OATMEAL WITH ALMOND BUTTER

**2 servings**
- *400ml (1 ⅔ cups) rice milk*
- *salt*
- *50g (¼ cup) gluten free oats*
- *1 teaspoon of almond butter*

STEP 1: Bring the rice milk to a boil. Gradually add the oats, stirring constantly, and let it simmer on low heat for 8 minutes. Stir frequently.

STEP 2: Pour the porridge into bowls and serve almond butter on a side.

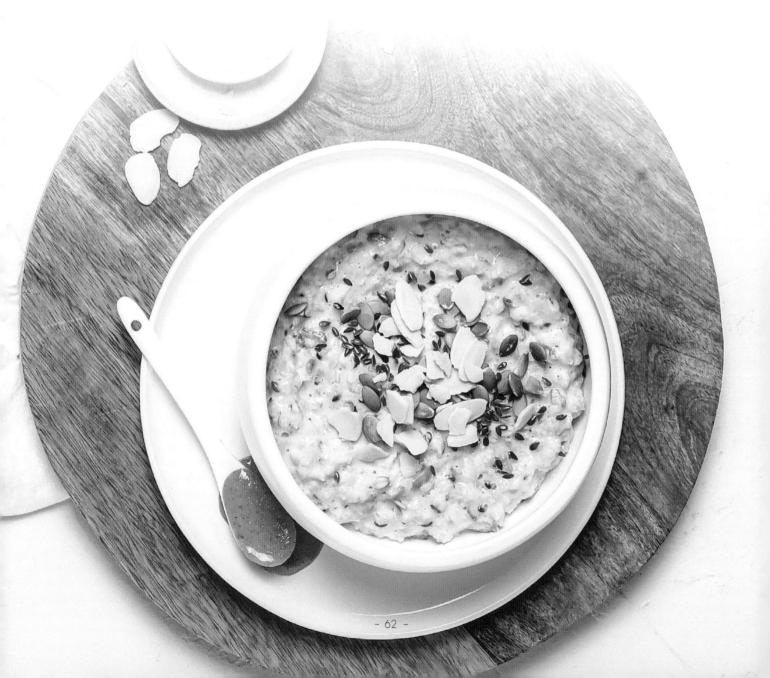

## VARIATIONS TO TRY:

YOGURT

Top porridge with 2-3 tabelspoons of sheep or goat yogurt or quark.

SEEDS AND BERRIES

Top with sliced almonds and seeds (pumpkin seeds and/or sunflower, lin/flaxseeds) or berries.

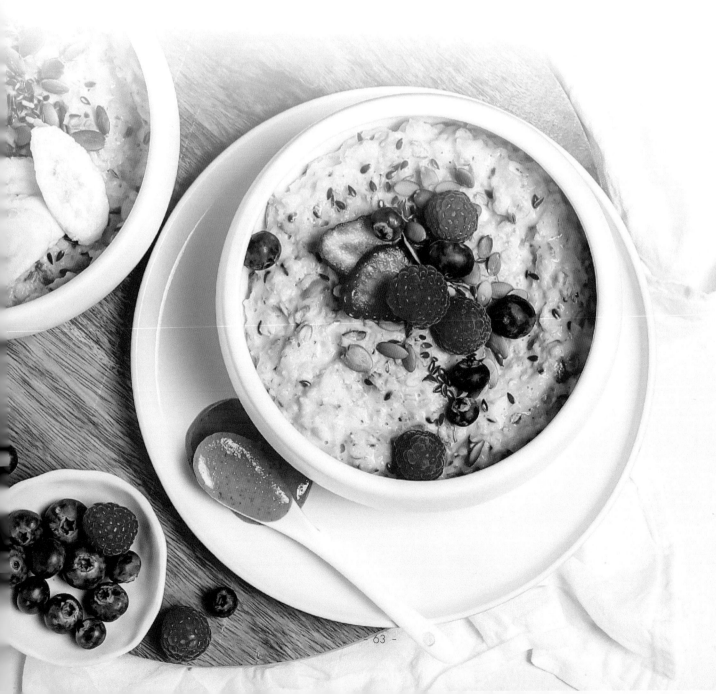

## 2.2. GLUTEN-FREE OVERNIGHT OATS

**2 servings**
- *3 tablespoons of gluten free rolled oats*
- *½ tablespoons of chia seeds*
- *75g (⅓ cup) plain full-fat sheep or goat yogurt*

STEP 1: Mix chia seeds and rolled oats with 125ml (½ cup) of water to create a liquid paste. Allow it to soak in the refrigerator overnight.

STEP 2: In the morning, combine the mixture with oil and yogurt and drizzle a few drops of honey on top.

### VARIATIONS TO TRY:

- Top with sliced almonds and pumpkin/sunflower seeds.
- Add assorted berries or banana slices.

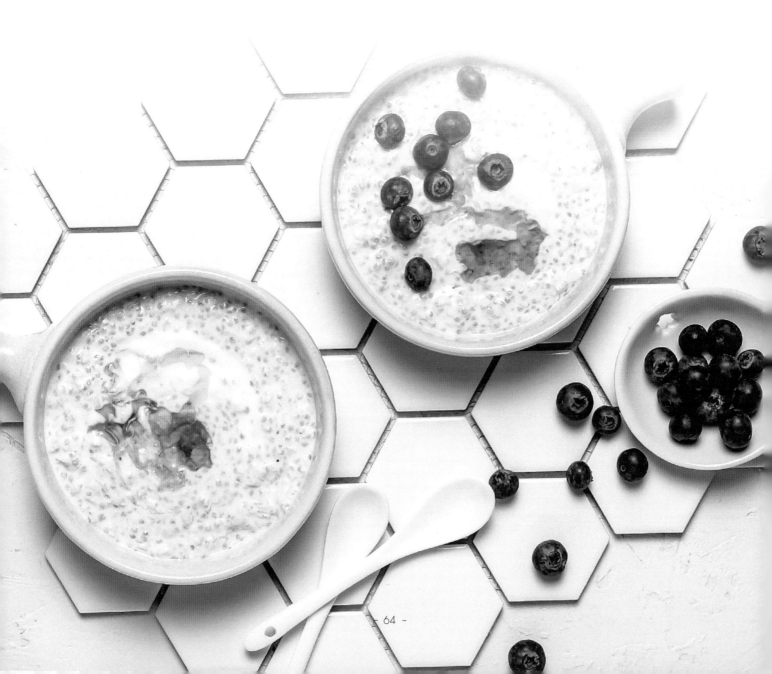

# 3. BLISS PARFAIT

**2 servings**
- 12 tablespoons of plain sheep yogurt
- touch of honey
- freshly squeezed lime juice
- flaxseeds, pumpkin seeds and/or
  sunflower seeds
- fresh mint leaves
- 2 tablespoons of extra virgin olive oil or
  flaxseed/linseedoil
- optional: 4 tablespoons of sheep quark
  (if available)

STEP 1: Combine yogurt, (optional: quark) lime juice, extra virgin olive oil or flaxseed/linseed oil, and honey in a blender.

STEP 2: Pour the creamy yogurt blend into a glass. Sprinkle with a mix of seeds and garnish with a fresh mint leaf.

## VARIATIONS TO TRY:
- Top with sliced almonds
- Add assorted berries

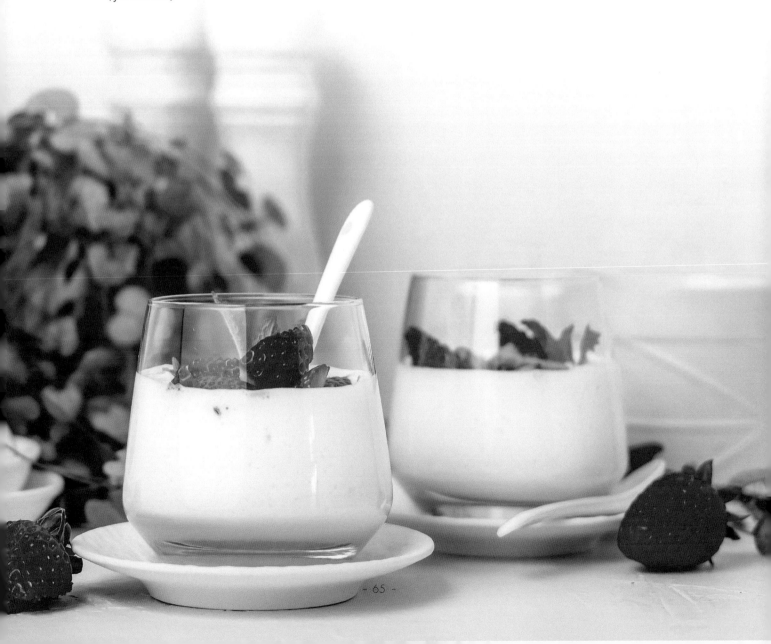

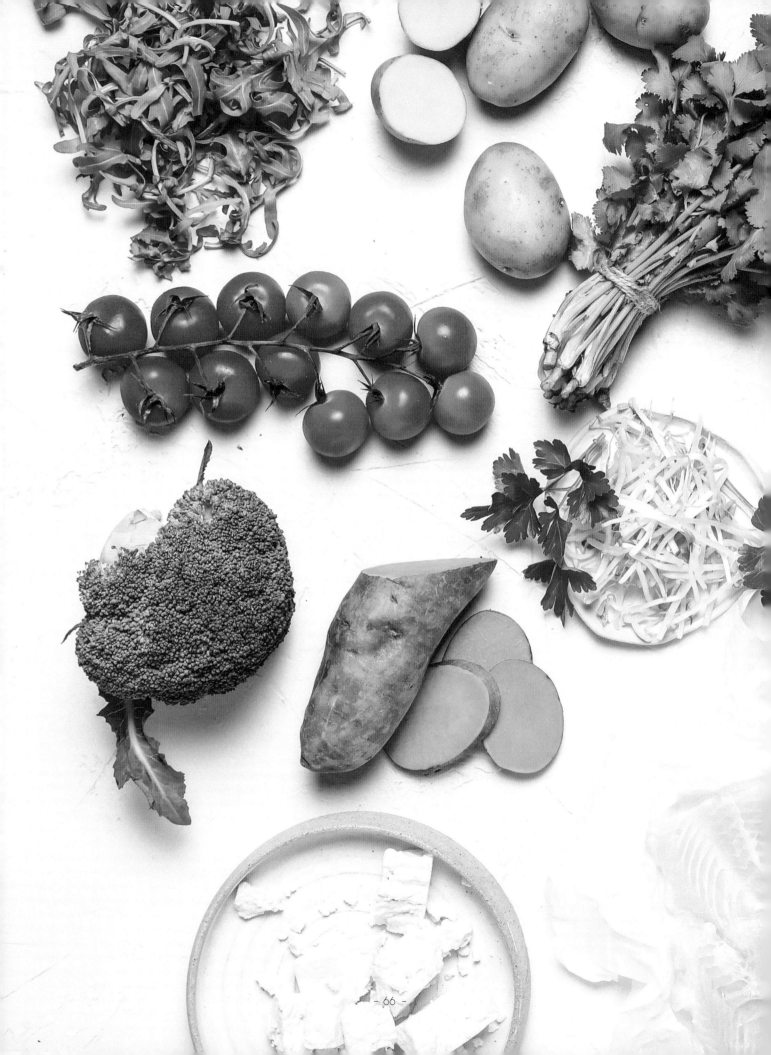

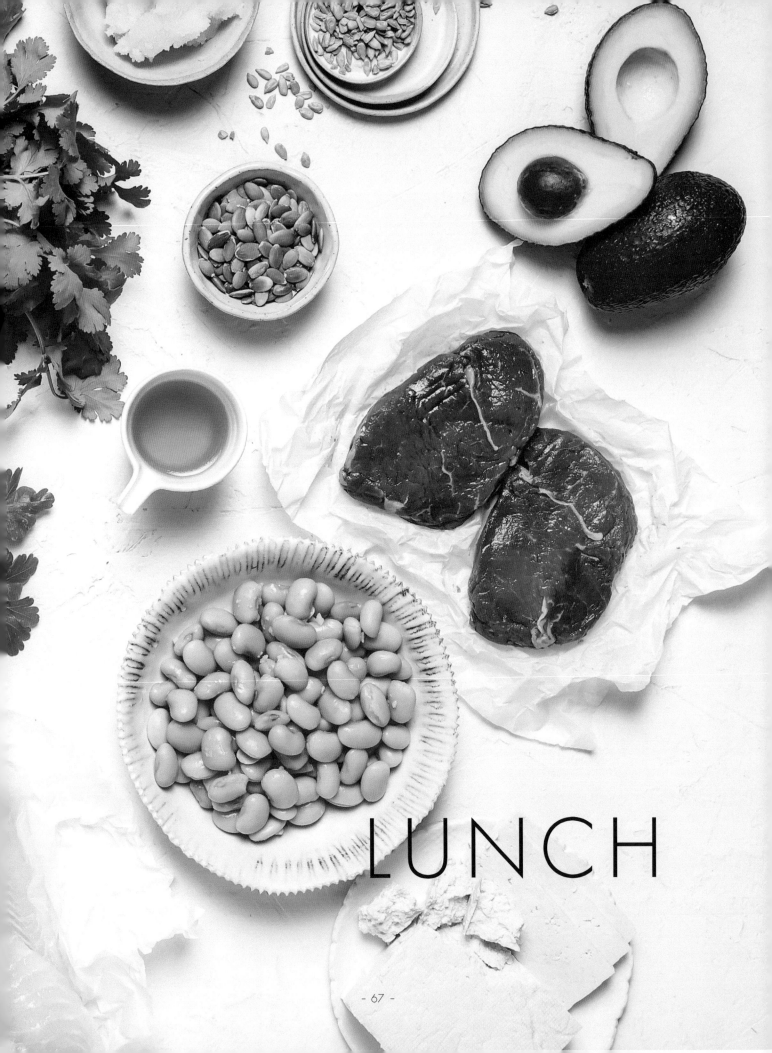

LUNCH

# 4. COOKED SEASONAL VEGETABLES

## 4.1. SEASONAL VEGETABLE MEDLEY WITH FETA

**2 servings**

• *1 zucchini*
• *2 big carrots*
• *250g feta cheese*
• *salt & pepper*
• *1 teaspoon of butter*
• *extra virgin olive oil*
• *fresh basil*
• *1 lime*

STEP 1: Using a vegetable peeler, cut the carrots and zucchini into narrow ribbons. Toss the vegetables in a bowl with salt and pepper, add a couple of small butter pieces.

STEP 2: Then place the vegetables in the steam tray. Set the steamer in a saucepan with just a little water so that the water doesn't touch the bottom part of the steamer. Steam on low heat for up to 8 minutes. Keep vegetables crunchy: aim for al dente veggies that are firm to the bite.

STEP 3. Arrange the vegetables on plates. Drizzle a little lime juice and olive oil on top. Garnish with basil leaves and top with feta cheese.

**TIP:** Feel free to use any seasonal vegetables you have on hand as substitutes.

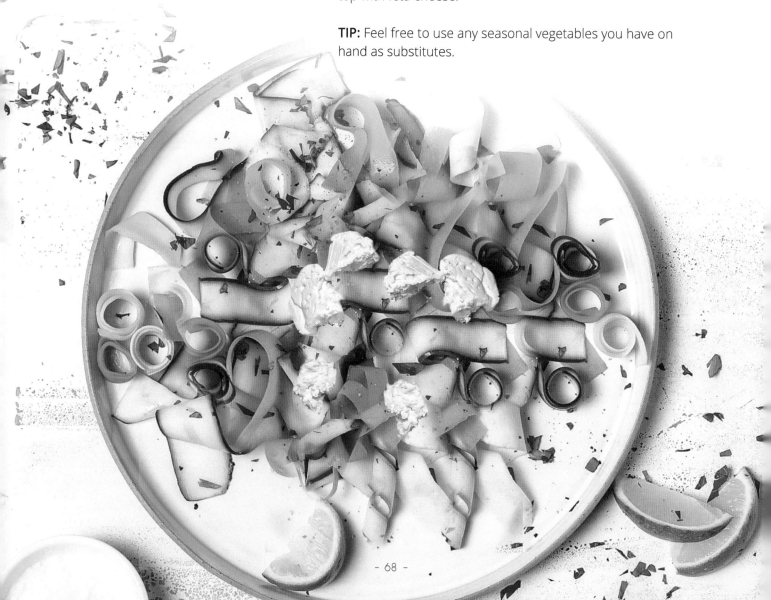

# 4.2. REFRESHING SEASONAL VEGETABLES AND POTATO MEDLEY

**2 servings**
- *1 teaspoon of ghee*
- *1 tbsp olive oil*
- *sea salt and freshly ground black pepper*
- *red chili flakes*
- *1 small cauliflower (or 1 bunch green asparagus or 1 small broccoli)*
- *8 cooked baby potatoes from the day before halved*
- *handful of scallions (also known as spring onions)*
- *optional side: 125 g (4 ½ oz) quark combined with 2 spring onions (or scallions) cut into rings, salt and pepper, red chili flakes.*

STEP 1: Cook the mini cauliflower or broccoli heads 6-7 minutes (or asparagus 2-3 minutes) in well-salted boiling water, remove and let drain. Keep vegetables crunchy: aim for al dente veggies that are firm to the bite.

STEP 2: In the meantime, heat the ghee in a skillet and fry the baby potatoes on all sides 3-4 minutes and season with a little salt, scallions.

STEP 3: Then transfer the vegetables to a plate and brush with a little olive oil. Serve with the baby potatoes and sprinkle with chili flakes.

Optional: add quark mixture as a side dish.

**TIP:** Feel free to use any seasonal vegetables you have on hand as substitutes.

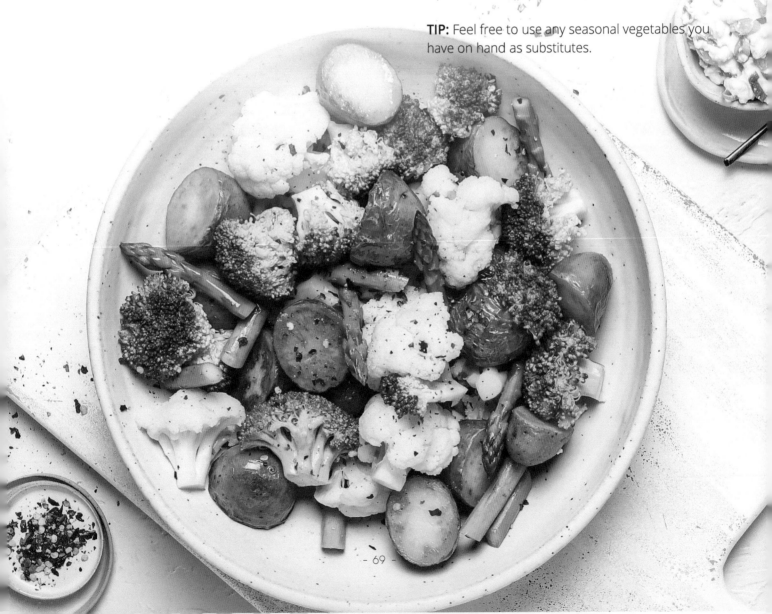

## 4.3. TANTALIZING ASPARAGUS WITH MEATBALLS

**2 servings**

- *1 teaspoon of Ghee*
- *1 bunch green asparagus*
- *200g (7 oz) minced veal*
- *1 egg*
- *25g (1 oz) pine nuts and few for garnish*
- *20g (½ oz) mustard*
- *100g (3½ oz) onions finely diced*
- *2 garlic cloves minced*
- *salt*

STEP 1: Place the asparagus in a skillet, add water, and cook with a pinch of salt for 2 - 3 minutes. Keep vegetables crunchy: aim for al dente veggies that are firm to the bite.

STEP 2: In the meantime, prepare the meatballs by mixing all the ingredients. Heat the ghee over medium-high heat, sauté the pine nuts (move them to a plate), and then gently cook the meatballs for 2-3 minutes on each side. Avoid browning!

STEP 3: Transfer the asparagus to a plate and drizzle with a touch of olive oil. Serve the asparagus with meatballs and garnish with roasted pine nuts.

**TIP:** Feel free to use any seasonal vegetables you have on hand as substitutes.

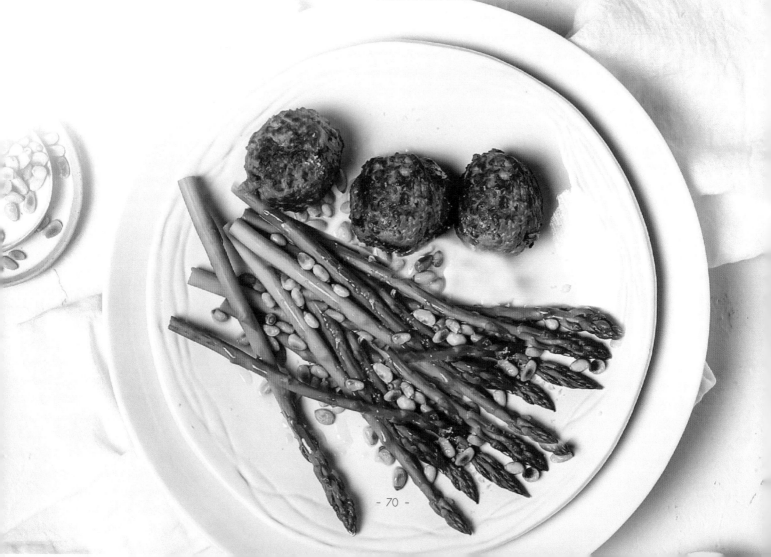

# 4.4. TOFU WITH RIBBON VEGETABLES

**2 servings**

- 250g tofu
- 100g (3½ oz) zucchini cut into narrow ribbons with vegetable peeler
- 100g (3½ oz) parsnip cut into narrow ribbons with vegetable peeler
- freshly squeezed lemon juice
- parsley
- salt & pepper
- 1 tbsp ghee
- extra virgin olive oil

STEP 1: In a skillet, heat the ghee over medium-high heat. Steam-Sauté tofu until golden. Do not brown!

STEP 2: In another skillet, heat the remaining ghee over medium-high heat. Steam-Sauté zucchini and parsnip with salt, pepper and fresh herbs until tender. Keep vegetables crunchy: aim for al dente veggies that are firm to the bite.

STEP 3: Place the tofu and vegetables on a plate with a garnish of fresh parsley. Drizzle with lemon juice and olive oil.

**TIP:** Feel free to use any seasonal vegetables you have on hand as substitutes.

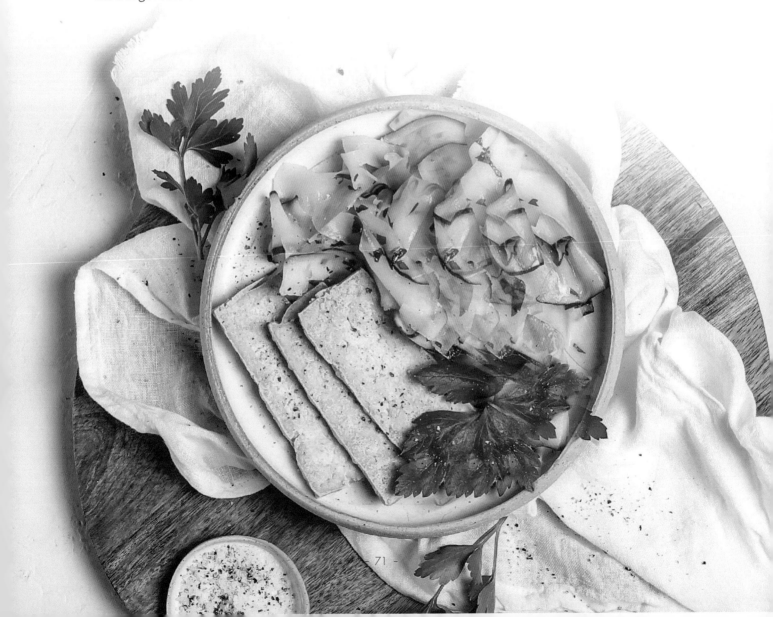

## 4.5. WILD SALMON WITH RIBBON VEGETABLES

**2 servings**

- 2 pieces wild salmon (125g (4½ oz each)
- 100g (3½oz) zucchini cut into narrow ribbons with vegetable peeler
- 100g (3½ oz) parsnip cut into narrow ribbons with vegetable peeler
- freshly squeezed lemon juice
- parsley
- salt & pepper
- 1 tbsp ghee
- extra virgin olive oil

STEP 1: Heat ghee in a skillet, sear the salmon for about 3 minutes on each side. Remove from heat and let it steam in the skillet.

STEP 2: In another skillet, heat the remaining ghee over medium-high heat. Steam-Sauté zucchini and parsnip with salt, pepper, and fresh herbs until tender. Keep vegetables crunchy: aim for al dente veggies that are firm to the bite.

STEP 3: Place the salmon with a garnish of fresh parsley and the steamed vegetables on a plate. Drizzle with lemon juice and olive oil.

**TIP:** Feel free to use any seasonal vegetables you have on hand as substitutes.

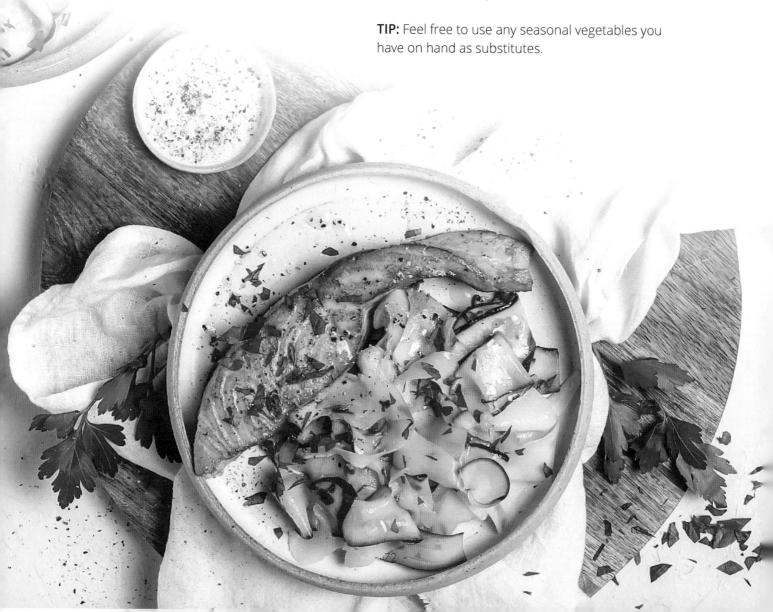

# 4.6. SAVORY PANCAKES WITH ARTICHOKE HEARTS

**2 servings**

## PANCAKES
- 1 tbsp ghee
- 50g (2 oz) coarsely ground spelt or buckwheat flour
- 1 egg
- 100g (3½ oz) sheep's milk sour cream
- 2 pinches of baking powder
- salt & pepper

## ARTICHOKE HEARTS
- 240g (8½ oz) artichoke hearts from a jar, halved
- handful of scallions (also known as spring onions)
- red chili flakes
- salt & pepper
- 1 tbsp olive oil

STEP 1: Combine sour cream, spelt (or buckwheat), egg, baking powder, salt and pepper to make a smooth batter in a bowl or blender.

STEP 2: In a skillet with heated ghee, cook small round pancakes on both sides until golden.

STEP 3: Heat the ghee in a skillet and sauté the artichoke hearts. After 1 minute, add the scallion rings and season with chili flakes, salt and pepper to taste. You can also serve this dish with your choice of other sautéed vegetables.

## VARIATIONS TO TRY:

- Breakfast Bliss: Pair pancakes with spreads, smoked salmon or other breakfast favorites.
- Dessert Delight: Top pancakes with a touch of mashed raspberry for a sweet treat.

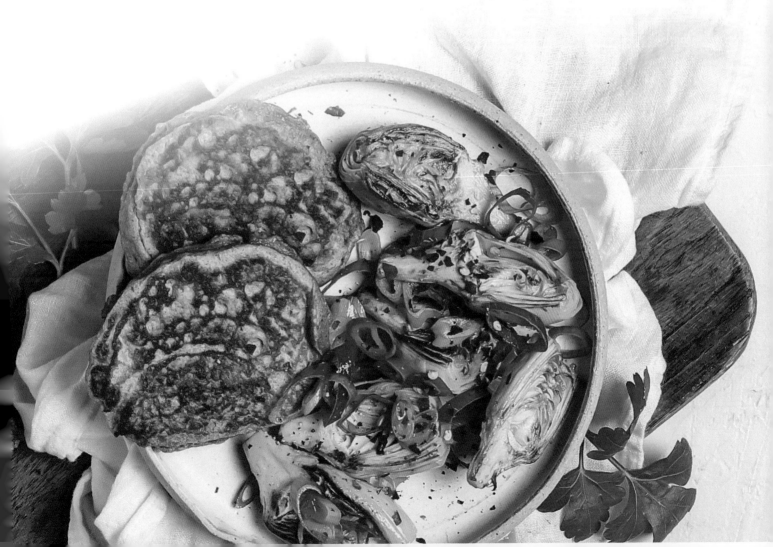

## 4.7. BEAN MEDLEY WITH SMOKED TOFU

**2 servings**
- 250g smoked tofu
- 1 onion cut into rings
- ½ hearted or pointed cabbage (~250g (9 oz) cut into thin strips
- 150g (5½ oz) white beans from a jar, rinsed and drained
- lime juice
- salt & pepper
- 1 tbsp ghee
- 1-2 tbsp balsamic vinegar
- 2 tbsp extra virgin olive oil
- fresh parsley

STEP 1: Heat ghee in a skillet. Sauté onions until softened. Add cabbage and cook covered for 1 minute. Stir in beans and season immediately with balsamic vinegar, salt and pepper. Mix and cook for an additional 2 minutes in the covered skillet.

STEP 2: In another skillet, heat the remaining ghee over medium-high heat. Sauté tofu until golden. Do not brown!

STEP 3: Place the tofu on top of the bean medley on a plate. Garnish with fresh parsley.

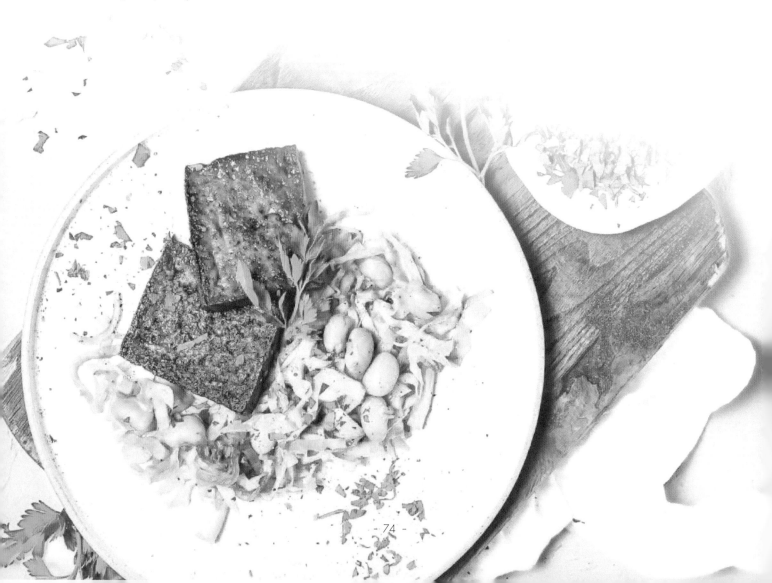

# 5. GLUTEN-FREE PASTA DISHES

## 5.1. BROWN RICE PASTA

### 2 servings

- *250g (9 oz) brown rice penne*
- *400 g (14 oz) chopped peeled tomatoes from a tin*
- *200g (8 oz) chickpeas from a jar*
- *40g (1½ oz) parmesan*
- *1 small yellow onion minced*
- *1 garlic clove minced*
- *fresh basil*
- *salt & pepper*
- *1 tbsp ghee*

STEP 1: Heat ghee in a saucepan, sauté onions and garlic. Add tomatoes, season and simmer covered for 6 minutes.

STEP 2: Rinse chickpeas and stir them into the sauce. Season to taste.

STEP 3: Cook pasta in well-salted boiling water until al dente. Drain and place on a plate. Pour tomato and chickpea sauce over pasta. Sprinkle with Parmesan and garnish with fresh basil.

### VARIATIONS TO TRY:
Choose from quinoa, lentil, chickpea pasta, or a blend of rice, corn and quinoa.

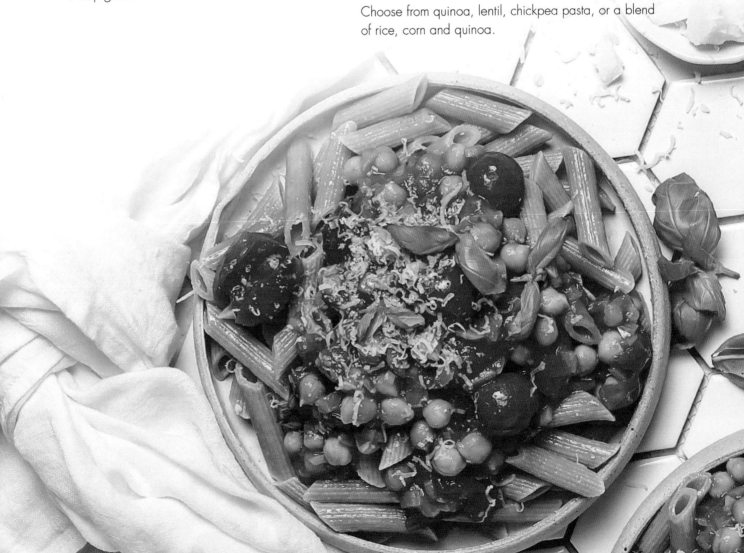

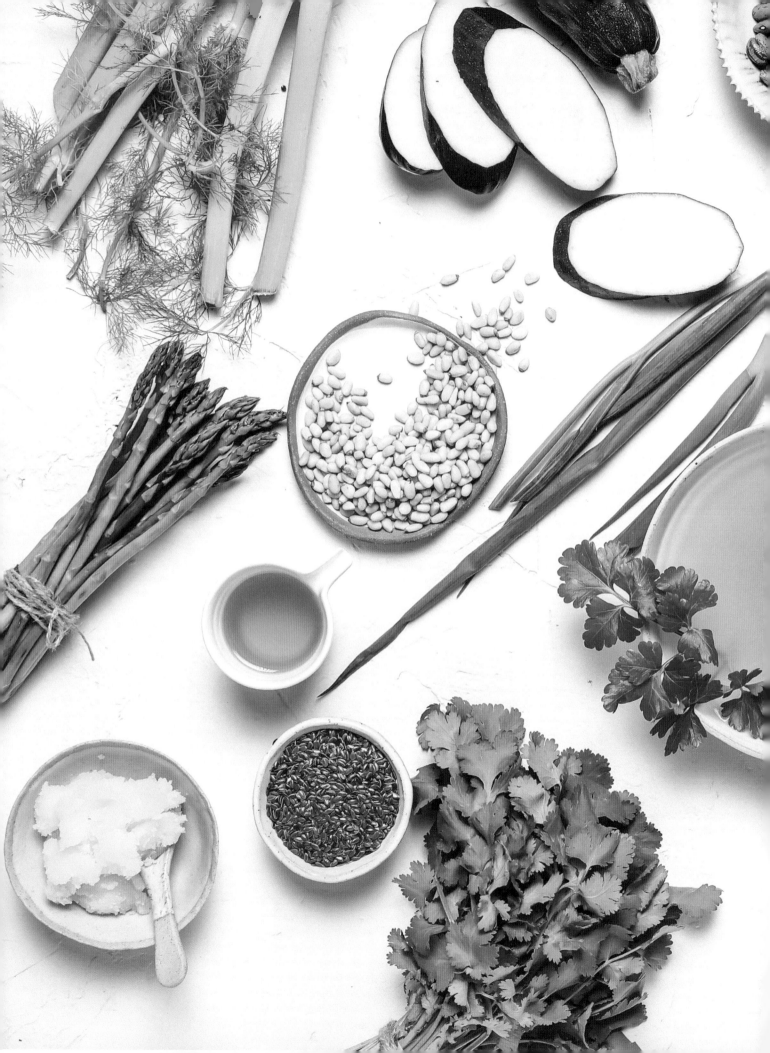

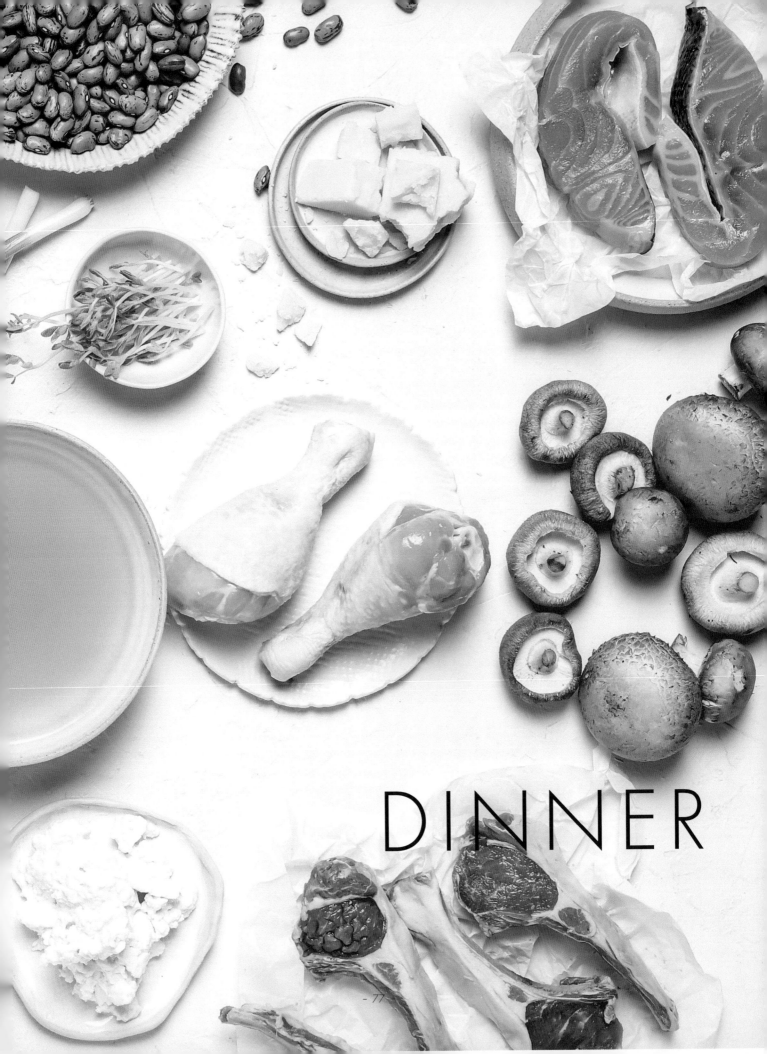

DINNER

# 6. VEGETABLE SOUPS

## 6.1 ENERGISING PEA SOUP

**2 servings**

- 1 tablespoon of ghee (clarified butter)
- 1 small yellow onion, peeled, halved and cut into rings
- 1 garlic clove, peeled, halved and minced
- 320g (11 oz) bag of frozen peas (petits pois)
- 500ml (17fl oz) vegetable broth
- ½ avocado, pit removed, peeled and cubed
- ½ handful of mint leaves, washed and coarsely chopped, plus few leaves for the garnish
- sea salt & freshly ground black pepper
- juice of 1 big or 2 small limes

STEP 1. Heat the ghee over medium-high heat and briefly sauté the onions and garlic. Do not brown! Add peas , stir well , pour in the vegetable broth and season with salt and pepper. Cook in a covered saucepan for 5 minutes.

STEP 2. In the meantime, combine the avocado cubes with the lime juice, a pinch of chopped mint and a little salt. Place in the middle of the plate and pour the soup on top.

STEP 3. Purée the soup well with the remaining chopped mint in a blender suited for hot foods. Place in the bowls and add mint leaves for garnish.

Optional: add a pinch of chili flakes to your taste.

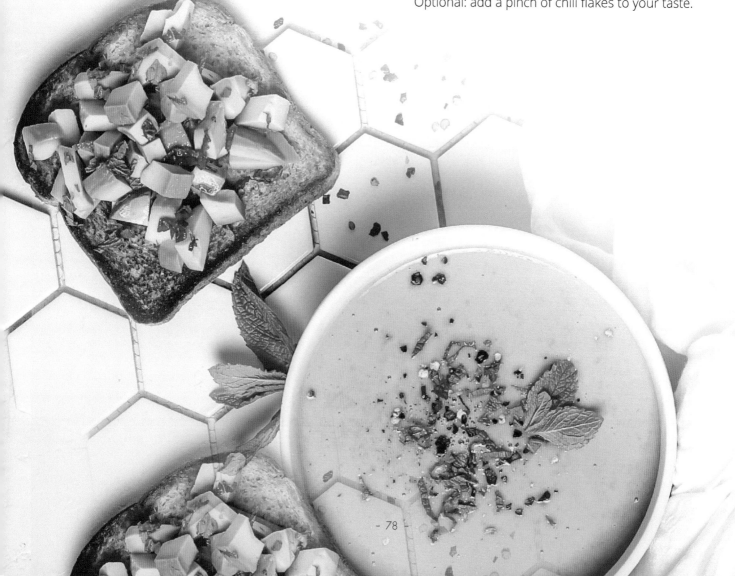

# 6.2 CALMING PUMPKIN SOUP

**2 servings**

- 1 teaspoon of ghee
- 1 small yellow onion, peeled and diced
- 1 garlic clove, peeled, halved and minced
- 1 small (340g / 12 oz) pumpkin washed, deseeded and cut into small pieces
- 500ml (17fl oz) vegetable broth
- 150g (5 ½ oz) coconut milk
- sea salt & freshly ground black pepper
- optional: add a pinch of curry and/or chili flakes to your taste
- 1 teaspoon of linseed / flaxseed or extra virgin olive oil for garnish

STEP 1: Heat the ghee over medium-high heat and briefly sauté the onions and garlic. Do not brown! Add the pumpkin pieces and spices you like (optional: pinch of curry and/or chili flakes), pour in the vegetable broth, add coconut milk and season with salt and pepper. Cook in a covered saucepan for 7-8 minutes.

STEP 2. Purée the soup well in a blender suited for hot foods. Place in the bowls and drizzle the oil on top with a sprinkle of spices and seeds.

STEP 3. Serve with gluten free crispbread or crackers.

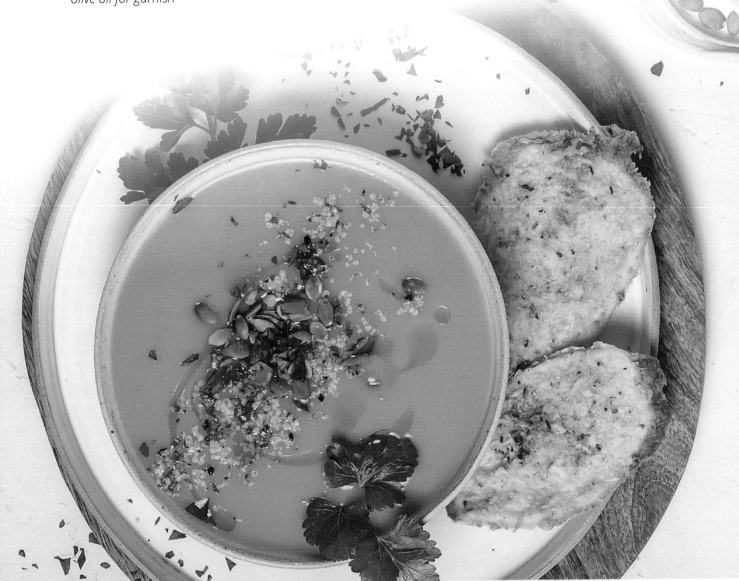

## 6.3. CARROT GINGER SOUP

**2 servings**

• 1 teaspoon of ghee
• 1 small yellow onion, peeled and diced
• 1 garlic clove, peeled, halved and minced
• 1 teaspoon freshly grated ginger
• 340g (12 oz) of carrots peeled, washed and
   cut into small pieces
• 500ml (17 fl oz) vegetable broth
• 150g (5½ oz) coconut milk
• sea salt & freshly ground black pepper
• 1 teaspoon of linseed / flaxseed or extra virgin
   olive oil for garnish

STEP 1. Heat the ghee over medium-high heat and briefly sauté the onions and garlic. Add the carrot pieces and ginger, pour in the vegetable broth, add coconut milk and season with salt and pepper. Cook in a covered saucepan for 7-8 minutes.

STEP 2. Purée the soup well in a blender suited for hot foods. Place in the bowls and drizzle the oil on top with a sprinkle of spices.

STEP 3. Serve with gluten free quinoa crispbread or crackers.

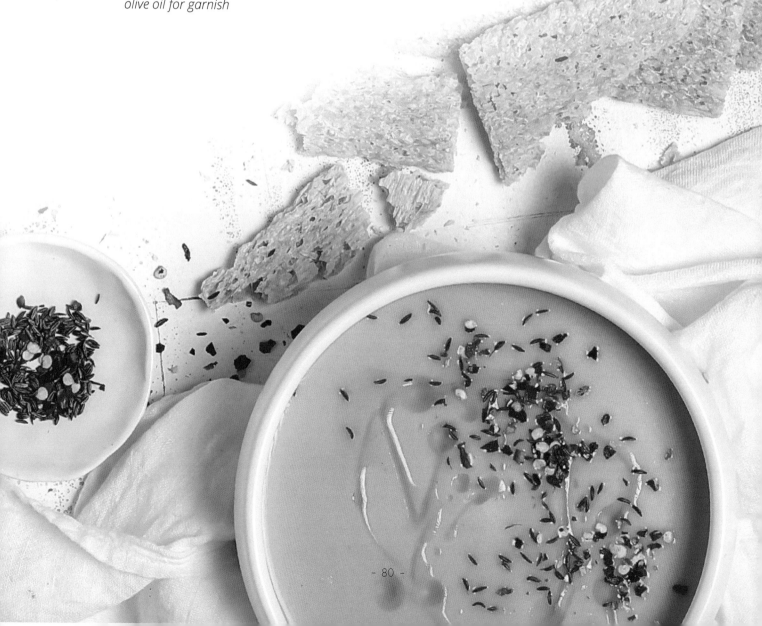

# 6.4. VITALITY BEETROOT SOUP

**2 servings**

- 1 tablespoon of ghee (clarified butter)
- 1 small yellow onion, peeled, halved and cut into rings
- 275g (9½ oz) cooked and peeled beetroot (purchased vacuum packed), cut into pieces
- 500ml (17 fl oz) vegetable broth
- sea salt & freshly ground black pepper
- parsley, dill
- 1 teaspoon of linseed / flaxseed or extra virgin olive oil for garnish

STEP 1. Heat the ghee over medium-high heat and briefly sauté the onions. Add the beetroot, pour in the vegetable broth and season with salt and pepper. Bring to boil in a covered saucepan and cook at a medium boil for 5 minutes.

STEP 2. Purée the soup well with chopped parsley in a blender suited for hot foods. Place in the bowls and drizzle the oil on top with a sprinkle of spices and garnish with parsley, dill.

STEP 3. Serve gluten-free toast with sheep/goat cheese spread (refer to breakfast spreads) beginning DETOX WEEK 2+.

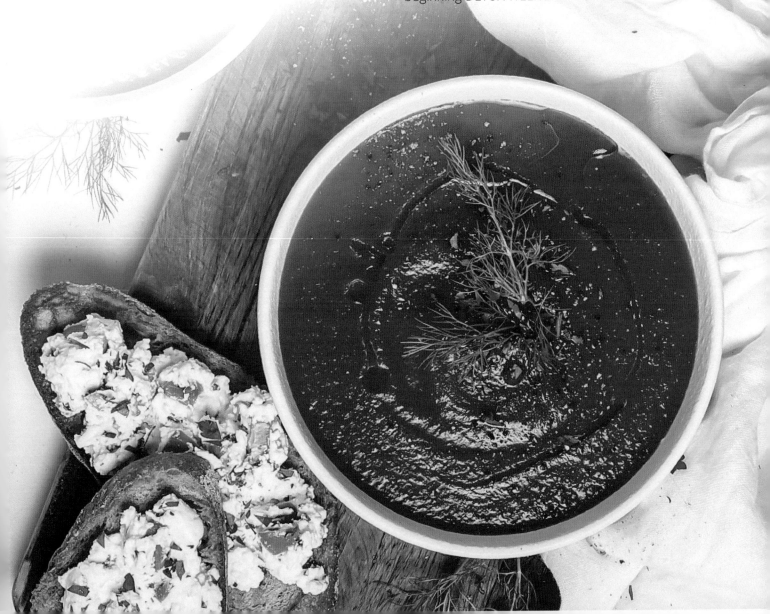

## 6.5. IMMUNE-BOOSTING MUSHROOM BOUILLON with FLATBREAD

**2 servings**

BOUILLON

• 1 tablespoon of ghee (clarified butter)
• 1 medium yellow onion, peeled and cut into thin strips
• 1 garlic clove, peeled, halved and minced
• 1 handful fresh champignons (or porcini mushrooms), rinsed off with cold water and chopped
• 500ml (17 fl oz) bone broth
• few coriander leaves
• sea salt & freshly ground black pepper

FLATBREAD

• sea salt
• 250g (9 oz) spelt flour
• 2 pinches bread seasoning
• 10g (½ oz) parmesan, grated

STEP 1. Heat the ghee over medium-high heat and briefly sauté the onions, garlic and fresh mushrooms. Pour in the bone broth and season with salt and pepper. Bring to boil in a covered saucepan and cook at a medium boil for 7-8 minutes. At the end of the cooking time, add coriander leaves.

STEP 2. Line a baking tray with parchment paper and preheat the oven to 230°C. Combine the flour with 2 pinches of salt and the bread seasoning, then add 230ml (8 fl oz) water. Stir until you have a creamy mixture. Use a tablespoon to thinly spread the mixture on the baking tray to form circles. Sprinkle the grated Parmesan on top and bake for 6-7 minutes.

STEP 3. Place the soup in bowls, top with coriander and serve with flatbread.

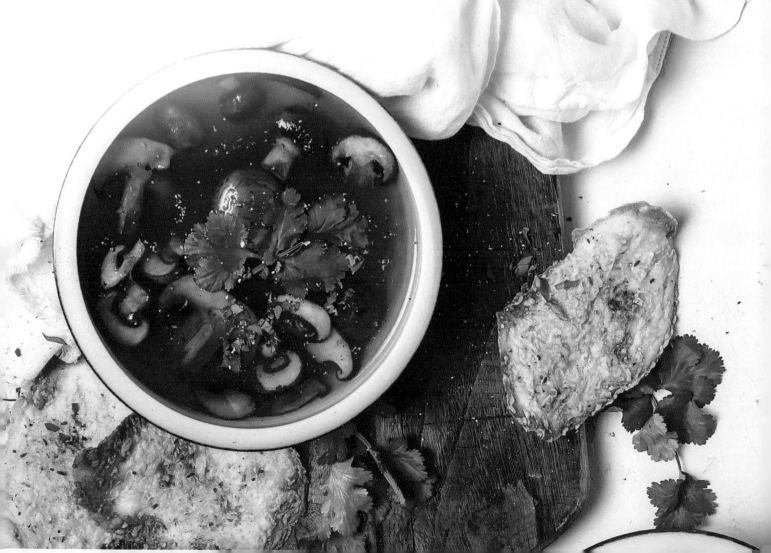

# 7. COOKED SEASONAL VEGETABLES

## 7.1. CHICKEN WITH SPROUTS & GREENS

**2 servings**

- *2 minute chicken (or beef filet) slices 50g (2 oz) each*
- *150g (5.3 oz) mung bean sprouts*
- *scallions (or also called spring onions)*
- *pesto*
- *½ red chili pepper*
- *lime juice*
- *salt*
- *1 tbsp ghee*
- *fresh coriander*

STEP 1: Heat ghee in a skillet. Sear the chicken (or beef filet) for 1 minute on each side. Season with salt and pepper. Remove from heat and let it rest in the skillet.

STEP 2: Sauté mung bean sprouts, spring onions and chili. Season with salt and a squeeze of lime juice. Cover the skillet with a lid and cook for an additional 2 minutes.

STEP 3: Place the filet slices on top of the vegetables on a plate. Drizzle pesto on the side of the filets and garnish with fresh coriander.

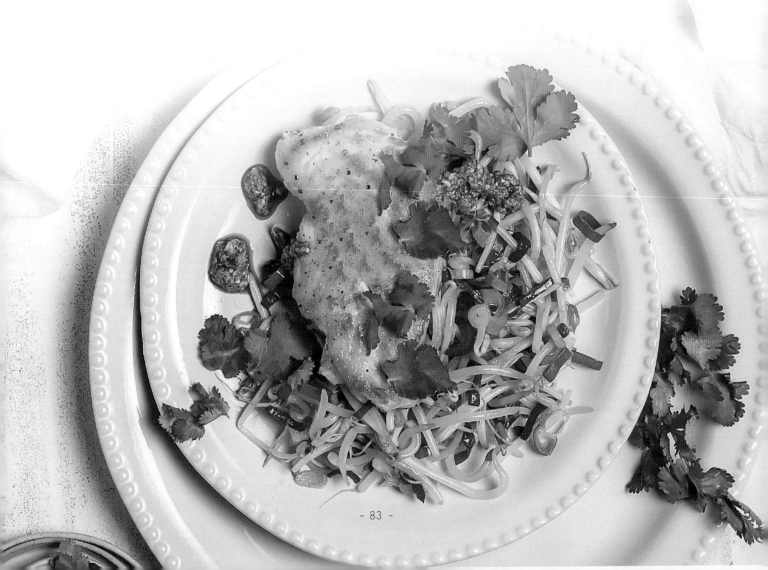

## 7.2. SOOTHING STEAMED FISH & VEGETABLES

### 2 servings

- 1 teaspoon of butter
- sea salt, freshly ground black pepper
- juice of ½ lime
- 100g (3½ oz) carrots
- 100g (3½ oz) parsley root
- 100g (3½ oz) zucchini
- 140g (5 oz) firm white fish filet (cod, hake, seabass, sole, or halibut)
- optional: basil

STEP 1. Place the white fish filet in the bottom part of a bamboo steamer or steam in the bag in an oven. Drizzle a couple of small butter pieces, sea salt and pepper on top of the fish.

STEP 2. Using a vegetable peeler, cut the carrots, parsley root, and zucchini into narrow ribbons. Toss the vegetables in a bowl with salt and pepper, add a couple of small butter pieces and then place them in the upper part of the bamboo steamer or steam in the bag in oven together with the fish (in separate oven bags). Set the steamer in a saucepan with just a little water, so that the water doesn't touch the bottom part of the steamer. Steam on low heat for up to 8 minutes. Keep vegetables crunchy: aim for al dente veggies that are firm to the bite.

STEP 3. Arrange the vegetables and fish on plates. Drizzle a little lime juice on top. Add basil for taste and garnish.

TIP: Feel free to use any seasonal vegetables you have on hand as substitutes.

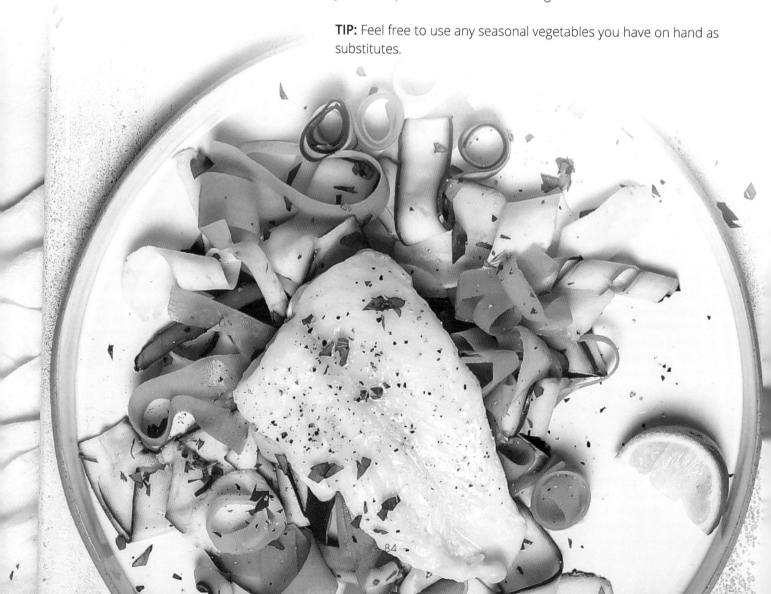

# 7.3. CHILEAN SEA BASS WITH BABY VEGGIE STIR-FRY

**2 servings**

- 2 pieces sea bass filet (125g / 4 oz each)
- 400g (2 cups) mixed baby veggies (e.g. carrots, leeks,turnip, sugar snap peas, zucchini etc.)
- 1 lime
- salt & pepper to taste
- 1 tbsp ghee (for cooking)
- extra virgin olive oil (for drizzling)
- fresh chives (for garnish)

STEP 1: Season the sea bass with salt and pepper on both sides. Heat the ghee in a skillet over medium-high heat. Sear the sea bass filets 2-3 minutes per side until golden and flakey. Remove and cover to keep warm.

STEP 2: In another skillet, heat the remaining ghee over medium-high heat. Toss in the mixed baby veggies and stir-fry for about 2-3 minutes until they are vibrant and slightly tender but still crunchy. Season with salt and pepper to taste.

STEP 3: Place the sea bass on a plate and spoon the stir-fried veggies alongside. Drizzle with fresh lime juice and a bit of olive oil. Garnish with fresh chives.

**TIP**: Feel free to use any seasonal vegetables you have on hand as substitutes.

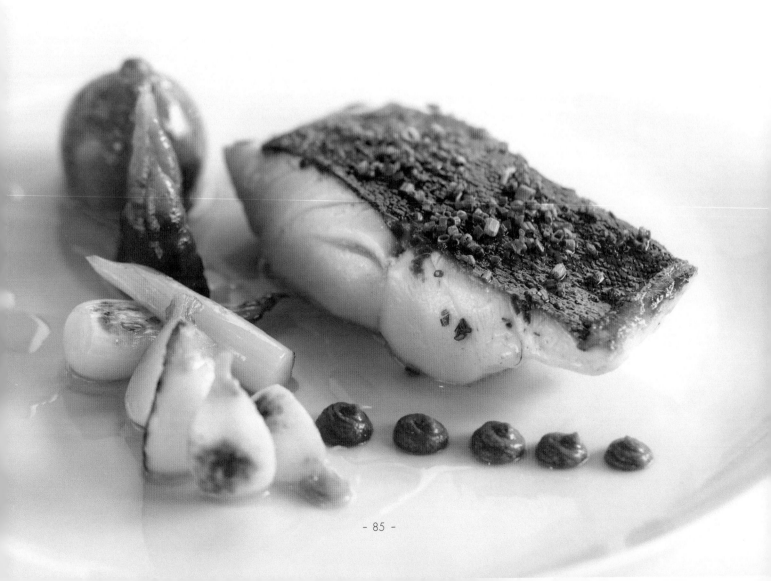

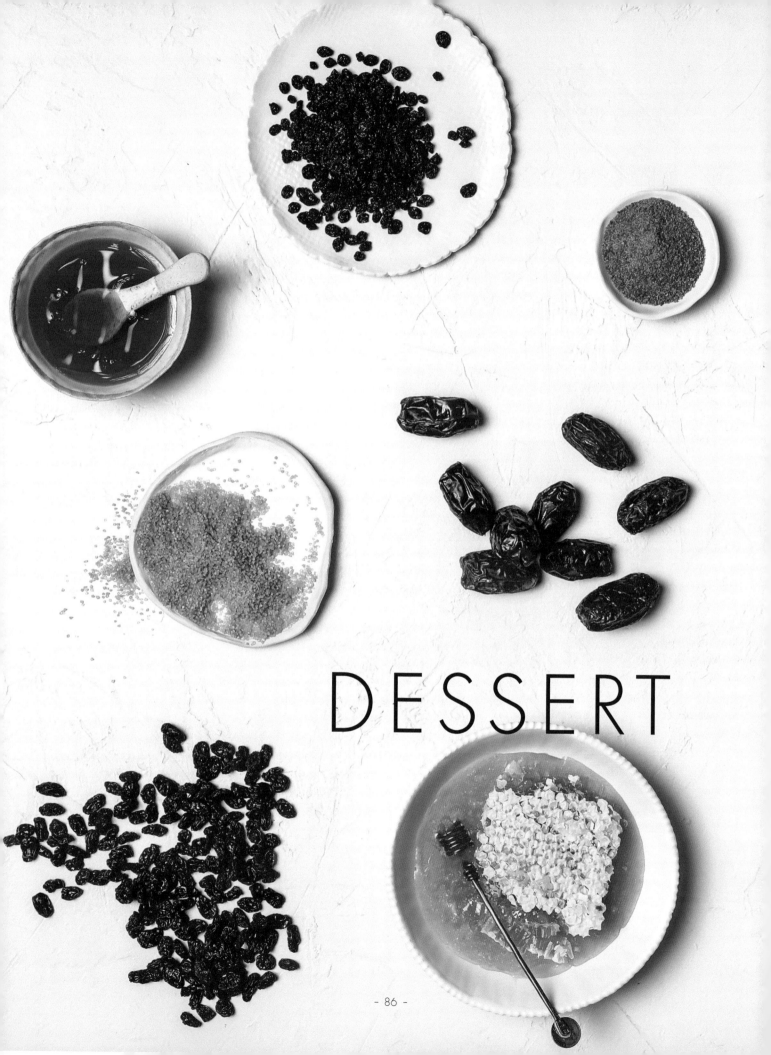

DESSERT

# 8. FRUIT FRENZY COMPOTE

**2 servings**

- 1 cup of apples, peeled and sliced
- 1 cup of pears, peeled and sliced
- ground cinnamon
- freshly squeezed lemon juice + zest
- fresh mint leaves
- optional: 1 teaspoon of honey

STEP 1: In a saucepan, combine sliced apples and pears with a touch of water. Squeeze lemon juice over the fruits, add honey, if desired, and a pinch of cinnamon.

STEP 2: Cook on low-medium heat, stirring occasionally, for about 7-8 minutes or until the fruits soften.

STEP 3: Remove from heat and let cool briefly. Just before serving, top the compote with a sprinkle of cinnamon, some lemon zest for a burst of color and garnish it with a fresh mint leaf.

## VARIATIONS TO TRY:

- Whip the heavy cream right before serving and add a dollop on top.
- Top with sliced almonds

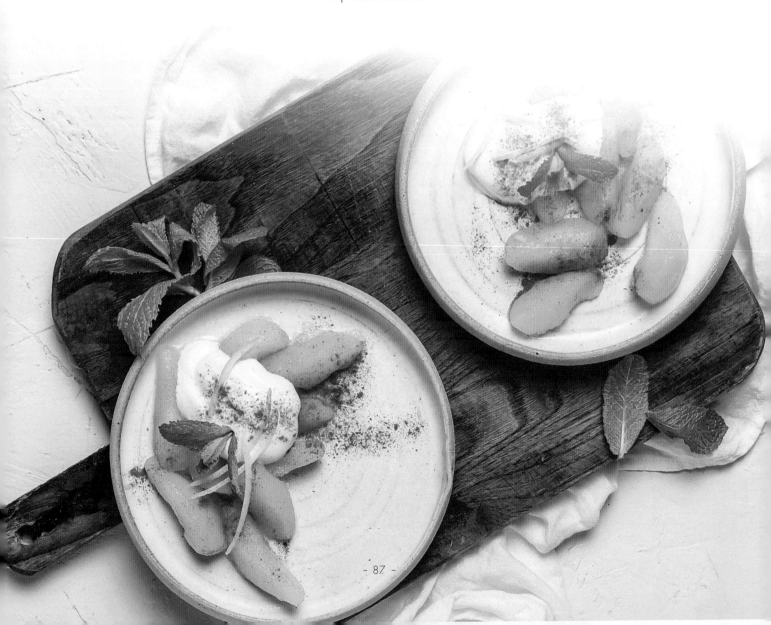

# 9. DARK CHOCOLATE RASPBERRY DELIGHT

**2 servings**

- *1 bar of 80% dark chocolate*
- *1 cup fresh raspberries*
- *fresh mint leaves*
- *12 tablespoons of plain sheep yogurt*
- *optional: 1 teaspoon of honey*

STEP 1: Mash raspberries (with honey if desired).

STEP 2: Layer yogurt and raspberry mash in glasses.

STEP 3: Top the raspberry sauce with fine dark chocolate curls or shavings. Garnish with a mint leaf.

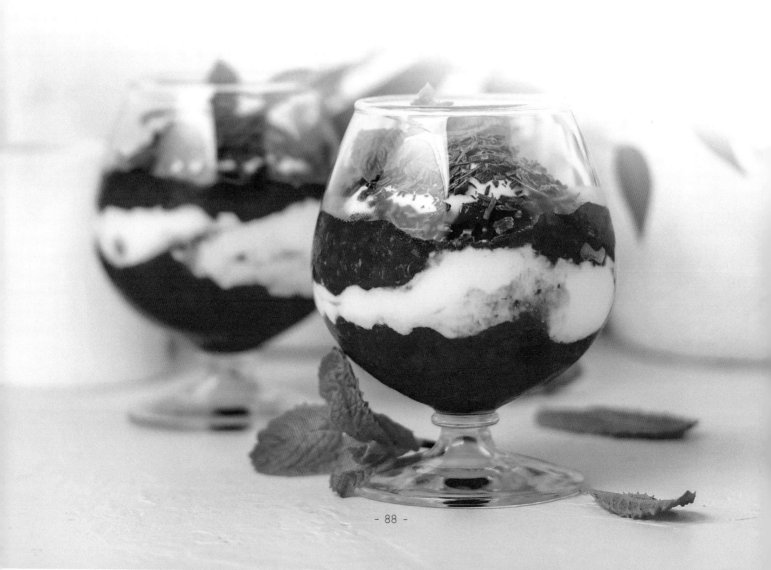

# 10. DARK CHOCOLATE MOUSSE

**2 servings**

- *1 bar high quality 80% dark chocolate finely chopped*
- *1 egg, room temperature*
- *1 cup (240ml) heavy whipping cream*
- *extra virgin olive oil*
- *sea salt*

STEP 1: Put the finely chopped chocolate and the egg in a blender. Add a pinch of sea salt and 2 teaspoons of extra virgin olive oil. Pour ¼ cup of boiling water onto the chocolate and blend at high speed until smooth.

STEP 2: Whip cold heavy cream to soft peaks, fold into chocolate mix until even, with no streaks. Adjust the texture to your taste by varying the amount of whipped cream used.

STEP 3: Divide the mixture into separate containers to your preferred serving size. Chilling is optional.

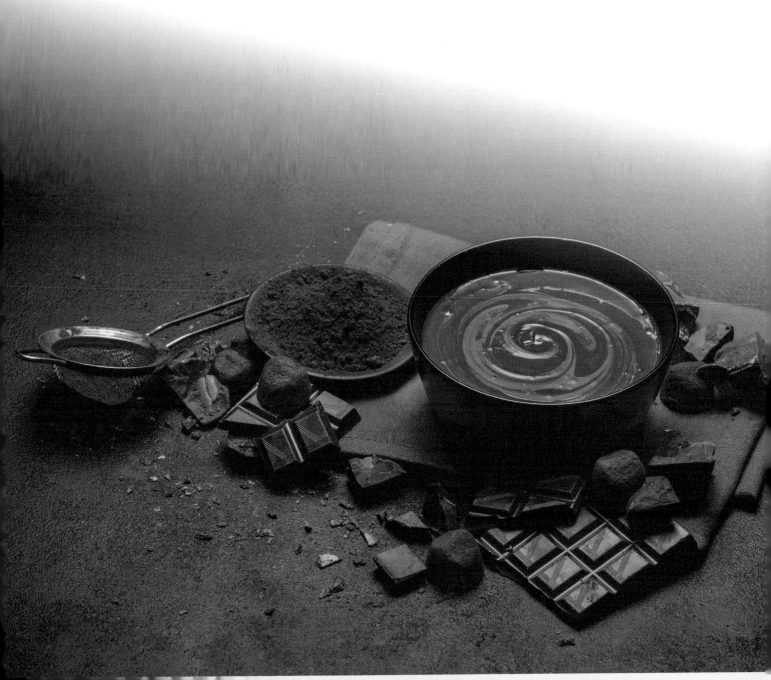

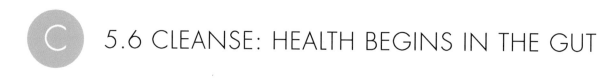

# 5.6 CLEANSE: HEALTH BEGINS IN THE GUT

## UNLOCK YOUR BODY'S HEALING POTENTIAL

A body free from toxins and excess acidity is primed to regenerate, revitalize and harness its innate self-healing abilities. The UPGRADERS® Method provides a blueprint for a clean lifestyle, enhanced by a specialized range of nutritional supplements, designed to detoxify the gut and boost the body's natural restorative functions. This aligns with the insights of F.X. Mayr:

*Toxicity in the gut leads to illness, accelerated aging and diminished attractiveness[39].*

*– F.X. Mayr*

Intestinal issues (caused by maldigestion) can lead to a range of noticeable and far-reaching symptoms such as, for example, feeling generally unwell, a lack of enthusiasm for work, mood swings, stress, depression, irritability, nervousness, foul breath, unpleasant body odor, a white-coated tongue, backache, sleep and vision problems, headaches, migraines, heart irregularities, morning dizziness, excessive perspiration, high blood pressure and joint pain, which may worsen with constipation.

Our bodies' vast microbial community plays a crucial role in digestion, mood, cognition, skin, heart, muscle, bone health, immunity and brain health, largely through the gut-brain axis and systemic interactions. This microbiome is essential for producing enzymes, vitamins and serotonin (the happiness hormone), underscoring its importance in immune function and overall well-being. However, age, antibiotics and unhealthy habits can negatively affect it. Embracing a lifestyle that includes interacting with a healthy, natural environment and consuming a diet free from harmful chemicals is vital for maintaining a vibrant microbiome. Avoiding detrimental agents like antibiotics and gluten is crucial to prevent conditions like leaky gut and Celiac disease, particularly when gluten is ingested alongside antibiotics.

By combining detoxification methods with a focus on nurturing the microbiome through a "Live dirty, eat clean!" approach, the UPGRADERS® method not only targets the detoxification and rejuvenation of the digestive system but also emphasizes the significance of a healthy microbiome for lasting health improvements. This holistic approach ensures an enhanced appearance and immune function and an improved quality of life with continued dietary and lifestyle practices supporting long-term benefits.

# ONLY A DETOXIFIED BODY CAN REGENERATE TO TRULY HEAL, LOSE WEIGHT, SLEEP BETTER, LOOK YOUNGER AND THRIVE

Chronic inflammation caused by toxic metabolites in the gut is the root cause of why we gain weight, develop chronic diseases and age faster.

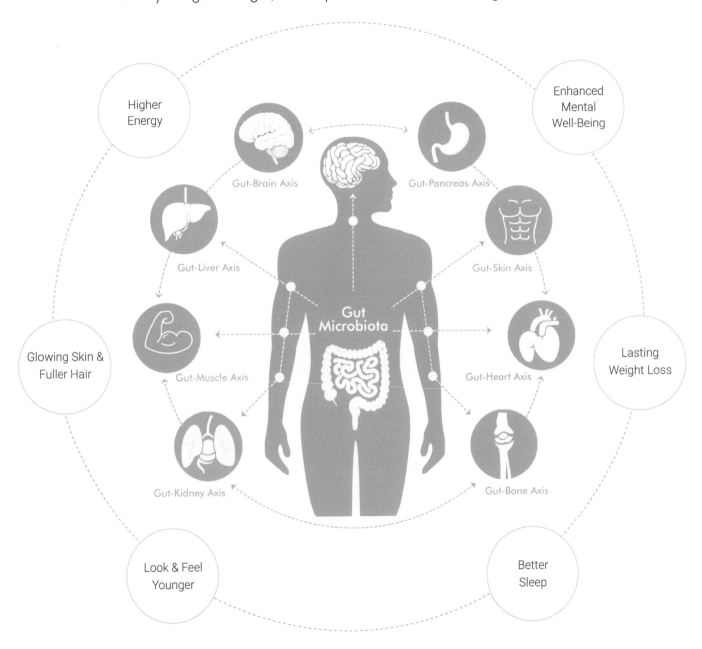

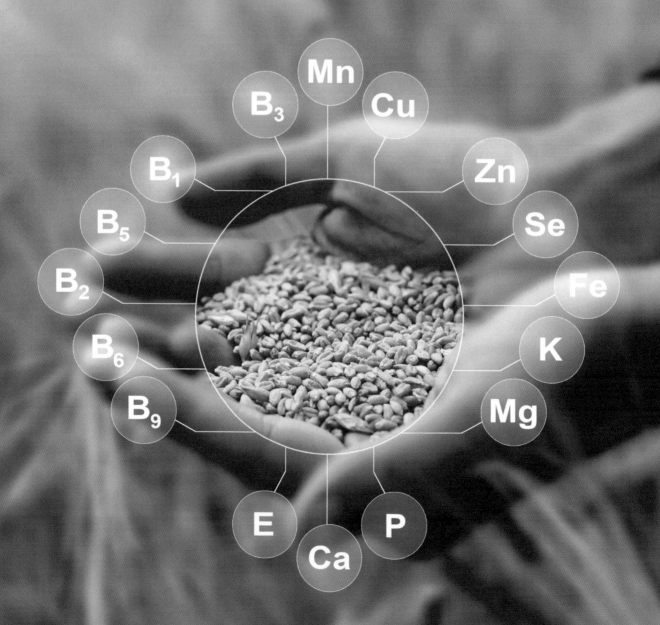

# 5.7 ENVIRONMENT: MINIMIZING TOXIN EXPOSURE

Improving our health and well-being significantly hinges on understanding our environment and minimizing toxin exposure. Simple changes can yield remarkable results.

**FOOD & DRINKS:** Antibiotics and growth hormones given to animals find their way into our food chain. Pesticides, artificial preservatives, flavors and colors can stealthily infiltrate our diet. Nutrient-rich local ingredients have been overshadowed by fast and processed foods, which often lack essential nutrients and contain harmful toxins. Soft drinks and many juices are loaded with concentrates and excessive sugar, contributing to metabolic health issues.

To minimize toxin exposure, prioritize fresh, locally sourced, organic and seasonal ingredients. Furthermore, carefully scrutinize product labels when making purchases. Eat plenty of green foods rich in chlorophyll to help cleanse the body.

**ALCOHOL & NICOTINE:** Excessive alcohol consumption elevates the risk of health conditions like liver or heart disease and bowel cancer. Tobacco smoke is loaded with thousands of chemicals, including 70 recognized carcinogens.

To reduce toxin exposure, practice moderation with alcohol and quit smoking.

**AIR & WATER:** Our tap water often harbors industrial, agricultural and pharmaceutical residues along with chlorine, hormones, heavy metals and pesticides. At the same time, pollutants from things like vehicle emissions and industrial waste, as well as indoor sources like air fresheners, scented candles and artificial room fragrances release harmful compounds into the air.

Prioritize a high-quality water filtration system. Opt for organic soy wax candles featuring lead-free cotton wicks or choose natural essential oil based air fresheners instead of synthetic diffusers, which may contain allergens capable of provoking skin reactions and eye irritation.

**PRODUCTS:** The average consumer uses approximately 10-30 products daily, unknowingly exposing himself to ingredients that can disrupt hormones and even cause cancer. Heavy metals such as aluminum in deodorants and lead in makeup are among these toxic substances. Moreover, our cleaning products often contain harmful chemicals.

Select all-natural, 'clean' products to lower toxin exposure. For 'Clean Life Certified' options without the worry of harmful ingredients, visit Upgraders.com.

# VI.CLEAN LIVING:
# YOUR JOURNEY BEGINS NOW...

## 6.1 MOVING FORWARD WITH BALANCE

After completing the **UPGRADERS®** 21-day Health & Beauty Pro DETOX & INTERMITTENT FASTING Program, it is crucial to smoothly transition back to regular eating. Continue applying the BALANCE lifestyle principles you learned during those 21 days. Don't forget to monitor your pH levels monthly to track acidity.

**DETOX 1-3 TIMES ANNUALLY:** For the **UPGRADES 21-day Health & Beauty Pro Detox & Intermittent Fasting Supplements**, visit upgraders.com or locate us on Amazon. Consider repeating the 21-day Detox program 1 to 3 times a year, as only a 'toxin-free' body can heal, lose weight, sleep better, look younger and thrive.

**SHARE THE ENTHUSIASM!** Now that you've experienced the incredible benefits of detox, why not spread the good news about your success to your family, friends, and co-workers? When you become an Affiliate Partner, your friends will enjoy an exclusive 11% discount on their orders, and you will receive a generous 10% commission. Visit our 'Become a Partner' page on upgraders.com to discover more about our Affiliate program and how you can spread the message about better health through BALANCE at all levels.

**PRIORITIZE GUT HEALTH:** Continue your wellness journey with UPGRADERS® supplements, meticulously crafted to uphold gut health as the foundation of holistic well-being. From digestion to mood, cognition, skin, heart health, muscle, bone strength, immunity and brain function, our products leverage the pivotal role of the gut, fostering comprehensive health from within. Explore our curated selection of 'Clean Life Certified' products on upgraders.com, committed to nurturing your body for lasting vitality.

Our 100% natural, highly concentrated supplements offer a perfectly balanced mix of bioactive nutrients and natural plant cofactors, ensuring superior bioavailability and effectiveness compared to synthetic vitamins.

**EXCITING UPCOMING LAUNCHES:** New! 'Clean Life Certified' Supplements, DIY Diagnostics and Inside-Out Skincare Line for Renewal and Rejuvenation. Crafted with top medical experts and naturopaths, these products meet the highest health standards.

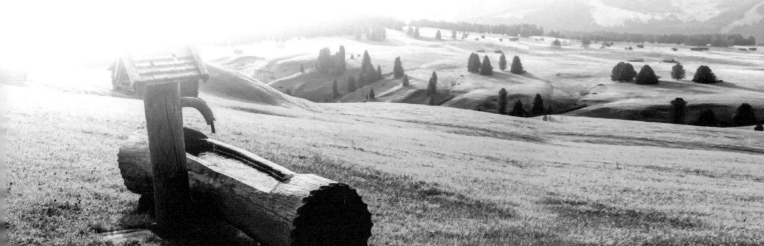

# 6.2 LET THE JOURNEY BEGIN ...

Experience the UPGRADERS® 'Clean Life' transformation. We firmly believe that a 'clean' body is the very foundation of health, beauty, vitality, and mental well-being. Our mission is to empower individuals across the globe in self-care, even amidst their busy lives, equipping them with the knowledge and the tools for the ultimate clean living experience. We're on a journey to redefine healthy living by blending timeless wisdom with cutting-edge technology. We delve deeply to address root causes, ensuring long lasting well-being and defying the passage of time.

The UPGRADERS® Method is not just a lifestyle; it's a resounding declaration that you deserve to live life to the fullest, reclaiming the very best version of yourself, while embracing the finest products and solutions proven to elevate your health. Choosing the Upgraders Method is an act of self-love. It is a journey of self-discovery, of healing and of growth. We are profoundly honored to take this transformative path with you.  We eagerly await the beginning of your remarkable journey. Together, we will forge a future defined by strength, beauty and well-being.

Welcome to an upgraded health and life — welcome to the extraordinary!

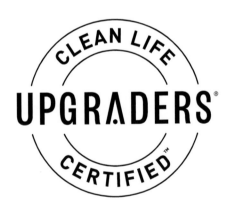

*Love,*

*Upgraders*

# REFERENCES

1. Claude Bernard, founder of modern Physiology, 1813-1878, cited in „Leçon sur les auto-intoxications dans les maladies" by Charles Bouchard 1885

2. Spivak I, Fluhr L, Elinav E. Local and systemic effects of microbiome-derived metabolites. EMBO Rep. 2022 Oct 6;23(10):e55664. doi: 10.15252/embr.202255664. Epub 2022 Aug 29. PMID: 36031866; PMCID: PMC9535759.

3. Sagar NA, Tarafdar S, Agarwal S, Tarafdar A, Sharma S. Polyamines: Functions, Metabolism, and Role in Human Disease Management. Med Sci (Basel). 2021 Jun 9;9(2):44. doi: 10.3390/medsci9020044. PMID: 34207607; PMCID: PMC8293435.

4. Nagpal R, Mainali R, Ahmadi S, Wang S, Singh R, Kavanagh K, Kitzman DW, Kushugulova A, Marotta F, Yadav H. Gut microbiome and aging: Physiological and mechanistic insights. Nutr Healthy Aging. 2018 Jun 15;4(4):267-285. doi: 10.3233/NHA-170030. PMID: 29951588; PMCID: PMC6004897.

5. Hughes RL, Holscher HD. Fueling Gut Microbes: A Review of the Interaction between Diet, Exercise, and the Gut Microbiota in Athletes. Adv Nutr. 2021 Dec 1;12(6):2190-2215. doi: 10.1093/advances/nmab077. PMID: 34229348; PMCID: PMC8634498.

6. Itoh et al., Peak blood ammonia and lactate after submaximal, maximal and supramaximal exercise in sprinters and long-distance runners.Eur J Appl Physiol Occup Physiol. 1990;60(4):271-6.

7. Mutch et al., Ammonia metabolism in exercise and fatigue: a review., Med Sci Sports Exerc. 1983;15(1):41-50.

8. Simons CC, Schouten LJ, Weijenberg MP, Goldbohm RA, van den Brandt PA. Bowel movement and constipation frequencies and the risk of colorectal cancer among men in the Netherlands Cohort Study on Diet and Cancer. Am J Epidemiol. 2010 Dec 15;172(12):1404-14. doi: 10.1093/aje/kwq307. Epub 2010 Oct 27. PMID: 20980354.

9. Ma N, Tian Y, Wu Y, Ma X. Contributions of the Interaction Between Dietary Protein and Gut Microbiota to Intestinal Health. Curr Protein Pept Sci. 2017;18(8):795-808. doi: 10.2174/1389203718666170216153505. PMID: 28215168.

10. Zhou ZL, Jia XB, Sun MF, et al. Neuroprotection of Fasting Mimicking Diet on MPTP-Induced Parkinson's Disease Mice via Gut Microbiota and Metabolites. Neurotherapeutics. 2019;16(3):741-760. doi:10.1007/s13311-019-00719-2

11. Hayaishi O. My life with tryptophan--never a dull moment. Protein Sci. 1993 Mar;2(3):472-5. doi: 10.1002/pro.5560020320. PMID: 8453383; PMCID: PMC2142392.

12. Ninan J, Feldman L. Ammonia Levels and Hepatic Encephalopathy in Patients with Known Chronic Liver Disease. J Hosp Med. 2017 Aug;12(8):659-661. doi: 10.12788/jhm.2794. PMID: 28786433.

13. Niknahad H, Jamshidzadeh A, Heidari R, Zarei M, Ommati MM. Ammonia-induced mitochondrial dysfunction and energy metabolism disturbances in isolated brain and liver mitochondria, and the effect of taurine administration: relevance to hepatic encephalopathy treatment. Clin Exp Hepatol. 2017;3(3):141-151. doi:10.5114/ceh.2017.68833

14. Bobermin LD, Souza DO, Gonçalves CA, Quincozes-Santos A. Resveratrol prevents ammonia-induced mitochondrial dysfunction and cellular redox imbalance in C6 astroglial cells. Nutr Neurosci. 2018 May;21(4):276-285. doi: 10.1080/1028415X.2017.1284375. Epub 2017 Feb 6. PMID: 28165879.

15. . MahmoudianDehkordi S, Arnold M, Nho K, Ahmad S, Jia W, Xie G, Louie G, Kueider-Paisley A, Moseley MA, Thompson JW, St John Williams L, Tenenbaum JD, Blach C, Baillie R, Han X, Bhattacharyya S, Toledo JB, Schafferer S, Klein S, Koal T, Risacher SL, Kling MA, Motsinger-Reif A, Rotroff DM, Jack J, Hankemeier T, Bennett DA, De Jager PL, Trojanowski JQ, Shaw LM, Weiner MW, Doraiswamy PM, van Duijn CM, Saykin AJ, Kastenmüller G, Kaddurah-Daouk R; Alzheimer's Disease Neuroimaging Initiative and the Alzheimer Disease Metabolomics Consortium. Altered bile acid profile associates with cognitive impairment in Alzheimer's disease-An emerging role for gut microbiome. Alzheimers Dement. 2019 Jan;15(1):76-92. doi: 10.1016/j.jalz.2018.07.217. Epub 2018 Oct 15. Erratum in: Alzheimers Dement. 2019 Apr;15(4):604. PMID: 30337151; PMCID: PMC6487485.

16. Itoh et al., Peak blood ammonia and lactate after submaximal, maximal and supramaximal exercise in sprinters and long-distance runners.Eur J Appl Physiol Occup Physiol. 1990;60(4):271-6.

17. Büngeler, W.: Die experimentelle Erzeugung von Leukämie und Lymphosarkom durch chronische Indol Vergiftung der Maus. Frankfurt. Z. Path. 44 (1933), 202

18. Li X, Zhang B, Hu Y, Zhao Y. New Insights Into Gut-Bacteria-Derived Indole and Its Derivatives in Intestinal and Liver Diseases. Front Pharmacol. 2021 Dec 13;12:769501. doi: 10.3389/fphar.2021.769501. PMID: 34966278; PMCID: PMC8710772.

19. González-Regueiro JA, Higuera-de la Tijera MF, Moreno-Alcántar R, Torre A. Pathophysiology of hepatic encephalopathy and future treatment options. Rev Gastroenterol Mex. 2019 Apr-Jun;84(2):195-203. English, Spanish. doi: 10.1016/j.rgmx.2019.02.004. Epub 2019 Apr 20. PMID: 31014748.

20. Senthong V et al. Trimethylamine N-Oxide and Mortality Risk in Patients With Peripheral Artery Disease. J Am Heart Assoc. 2016; 5:e004237

21. https://www.biovis-diagnostik.eu/wp-content/uploads/biovis-TMAO-DE.pdf

22. Makrecka-Kuka M, Volska K, Antone U, Vilskersts R, Grinberga S, Bandere D, Liepinsh E, Dambrova M. Trimethylamine N-oxide impairs pyruvate and fatty acid oxidation in cardiac mitochondria. Toxicol Lett. 2017 Feb 5;267:32-38. doi: 10.1016/j.toxlet.2016.12.017. Epub 2016 Dec 31. PMID: 28049038.

23. Alzheimer's & Dementia: The Journal of the Alzheimer's Association 2019 15, 76-92DOI: (10.1016/j.jalz.2018.07.217)

24. Sato, Y., Atarashi, K., Plichta, D.R. et al. Novel bile acid biosynthetic pathways are enriched in the microbiome of centenarians. Nature (2021 July 29th). https://doi.org/10.1038/s41586-021-03832-5

25. Lamichhane S, Sen P, Dickens AM, Orešič M, Bertram HC. Gut metabolome meets microbiome: A methodological perspective to understand the relationship between host and microbe. Methods. 2018 Oct 1;149:3-12. doi: 10.1016/j.ymeth.2018.04.029. Epub 2018 Apr 30. PMID: 29715508.

26. Binienda A, Twardowska A, Makaro A, Salaga M. Dietary Carbohydrates and Lipids in the Pathogenesis of Leaky Gut Syndrome: An Overview. Int J Mol Sci. 2020 Nov 8;21(21):8368. doi: 10.3390/ijms21218368. PMID: 33171587; PMCID: PMC7664638.

27. Harry Sokol et al. „Faecalibacterium prausnitzii is an anti-inflammatory commensal bacterium identified by gut microbiota analysis of Crohn disease patients", PNAS 2008 105:16731-16736

28. Dr. sc. med. Bodo Kuklinski. „Mitochondrien." iBooks 2015, ISBN EBook 978-3-89901-928-5

29. Goyal, M, Singh S, Sibinga E, Gould N, Rowland-Seymour A, Sharma R, Berger Z, Sleicher D, Maron D, Shihab H, Ranasinghe P, Linn S, Saha S, Bass E, Haythornthwaite J. Meditation programs for psychological stress and well-being. JAMA Intern Med. 2014 Mar; 174(3):357-68. doi:10.1001/jamainternmed.2013.13018; PMID: 24395196; PMCID: PMC4142584 https://pubmed.ncbi.nlm.nih.gov/24395196/

30. Orme-Johnson D, Barnes V. Effects of the transcendental meditation technique on trait anxiety. J Altern Complement Med. 2014 May;20(5):330-41. doi:10.1089/acm.2013.0204; PMID: 24107199

https://pubmed.ncbi.nlm.nih.gov/24107199/

31. Hofmann S, Gomez A. Mindfulness-Based Interventions for Anxiety and Depression. Psychiatr Clin North Am. 2017 Dec; 40(4):739-749. doi: 10.1016/j.psc.2017.08.008. PMID: 29080597; PMCID: PMC5679245. https://www.ncbi.nlm.nih.gov/pmc/articles/PMC5679245/

32. Ong J, Manber R, Segal Z, Xia Y, Shapiro S, Wyatt J. A Randomized Controlled Trial of Mindfulness Meditation for Chronic Insomnia. Sleep, Volume 37, Issue 9, 1 September 2014, Pages 1553 – 1563 https://doi.org/10.5665/sleep.4010

33. Garatachea N, Pareja-Galeano H, Sanchis-Gomar F, et al. Exercise attenuates the major hallmarks of aging. Rejuvenation Res. 2015;18(1):57-89. doi:10.1089/rej.2014.1623

34. Dimitrov S, Hulteng E, Hong S. Inflammation and exercise. Brain, Behavior, and Immunity. Volume 61, March 2017. Pages 60-68. https://doi.org/10.1016/j.bbi.2016.12.017

35. Tucker L. Physical activity and telomere length in U.S. men and women: An NHANES investigation. Preventative Medicine. Volume 100, July 2017, Pages 145-151 https://doi.org/10.1016/j.ypmed.2017.04.027

36. Eugene A, Masiak J. The Neuroprotective Aspects of Sleep. MEDtube Sci. 2015 Mar; 3(1): 35-40. PMID: 26594659; PMCID: PMC4651462 https://www.ncbi.nlm.nih.gov/pmc/articles/PMC4651462/

37. Vyazovskiy V. Sleep, recovery, and metaregulation: explaining the benefits of sleep. Nat Sci Sleep. 2015; 7: 171 – 184. doi: 10.2147/NSS.S54036; PMID: 26719733; PMCID: PMC4689288.

38. Walker, M. (2018). Why we sleep. Penguin Books.

39. Rauch, Erich. "Health Through Inner Body Cleansing" Seventh Edition. Thieme, Stuttgart 2017.

# ABOUT THE AUTHORS

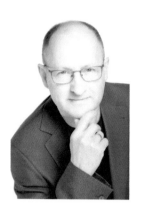

### DR. MED. HENNING SARTOR, PHD  - A Journey from Patient to Pioneer

Born in 1958 in Germany, Dr. Henning Sartor's unique path in medicine began after his initial training as an electronics technician, bringing a physicist's perspective to the natural sciences and medicine. His doctoral research in Clinical Chemistry at the University of Giessen laid the foundation for a career characterized by a deep dive into the causality of diseases.

Battling personal health challenges such as allergies, atopic dermatitis, and asthma, Dr. Sartor was driven to explore natural, foundational, and long-term treatments across the spectrum of medical conditions. His work in a bustling general practice directed his focus on chronic disease, particularly the critical roles of the gut microbiome and metabolic processes in health.

Through innovative diagnostic and therapeutic approaches, Dr. Sartor not only reclaimed his health but also provided groundbreaking solutions for patients wearied by traditional treatments. His extensive practical experience, coupled with contributions to scientific research, has yielded numerous publications and textbooks.

Today, esteemed within the Mayr medical community across Austria, Germany, and Switzerland, and serving as an educator at both the BIOVIS Academy and Lanserhof Academy, Dr. Sartor dedicates himself to disseminating his deep knowledge. The Upgraders method, a culmination of his personal and professional journey to achieving health balance, stands as a testament to his dedication to bringing comprehensive health restoration insights to people worldwide.

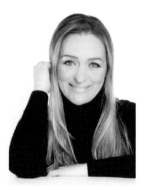

### HELEN M. LOORENTS, MBA  - From Healthcare Executive to Wellness Innovator

Founder & CEO of UPGRADERS®
Health & Wellness Coach, Nutritionist

Helen M. Loorents's story begins in Estonia and evolves across the USA, where she spent over 26 years in leadership roles at healthcare giants like GlaxoSmithKline, Johnson & Johnson, and Colgate. In these positions, Helen refined her search for healing solutions that align with the body's natural processes. Confronted with her own sensitivities to chemicals and the side effects of conventional medicine, she was driven to explore more gentle, natural ways to heal. Her deep dive into natural medicine and understanding the root causes of diseases led Helen to become a licensed health coach, nutritionist, Mayr-trained practitioner, and author. She advocates for a natural and holistic health paradigm that aims to treat the underlying causes of illness, not just the symptoms.

From a young age, Helen's heightened sensitivity to toxins guided her through significant challenges, especially during a crucial period in New York. There, amidst burnout and continuous health struggles, she turned to a renowned Alpine wellness clinic for refuge. The profound detoxification and healing she underwent there ignited a vision: to democratize such transformative wellness experiences. Motivated to replicate the clinic's holistic benefits for home practice, Helen developed a method that is both accessible and practical.

Fueled by a passion to share her knowledge, Helen founded UPGRADERS®. This venture is a testament to her commitment to disseminate a validated detox methodology and the ethos of clean living to a global audience. Helen's ambition is revolutionary—seeking to transform healthcare by promoting prevention and prioritizing natural remedies within a holistic health framework.

# ACKNOWLEDGEMENTS

We extend our deepest gratitude to Dr. Claudia Preyer, a distinguished Viennese surgeon whose expertise in root-cause healing and reconstructive approaches has been invaluable. Her meticulous attention to detail, coupled with her fluency in both English and German and her training as a Mayr doctor, were instrumental in bringing the Upgraders Method to the world. Dr. Preyer's dual perspective as both a doctor and a patient has fundamentally shaped our approach.

We also express our sincere appreciation to designer Külli Tõnisson (BrandAbout design agency) for her patience, flexibility, and creative vision, which have enriched this project immensely.

To my family and friends, your belief in me has been a source of unwavering support. Additionally, we thank the International Society of Mayr Doctors for three years of enlightening education and Lanserhof Clinic, whose healing services provided the insight that ignited our mission to heal the world one person at a time, naturally.

Our journey would not have been possible without the contributions of each of these remarkable individuals and organizations.

*Helen Marie Loorents,*

THE FOUNDER OF UPGRADERS

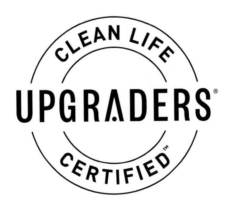

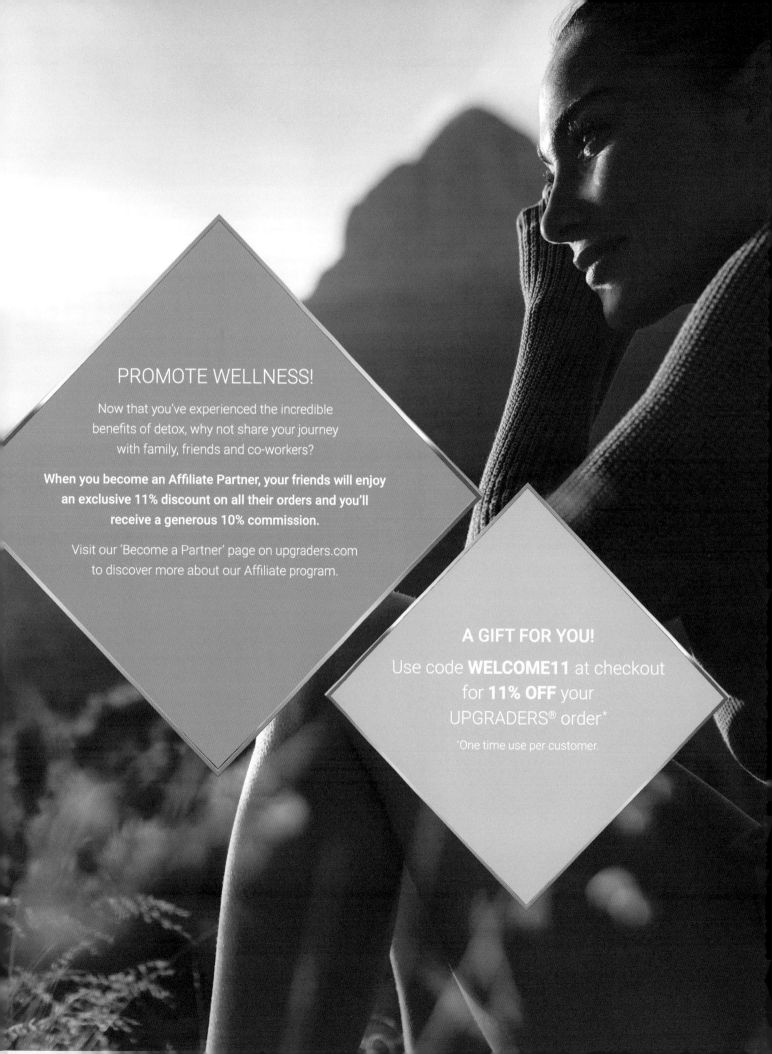

## PROMOTE WELLNESS!

Now that you've experienced the incredible benefits of detox, why not share your journey with family, friends and co-workers?

**When you become an Affiliate Partner, your friends will enjoy an exclusive 11% discount on all their orders and you'll receive a generous 10% commission.**

Visit our 'Become a Partner' page on upgraders.com to discover more about our Affiliate program.

## A GIFT FOR YOU!

Use code **WELCOME11** at checkout for **11% OFF** your UPGRADERS® order*

*One time use per customer.

Printed in Great Britain
by Amazon

49130435R00057